CW00429449

# Fixed and Removable Prosthodontics

**C. W. Barclay** BDS FDSRCPS DRD MRD
Lecturer, Prosthetic Dentistry, School of Dentistry,
The University of Birmingham, UK

**A. D. Walmsley** BDS MSc PhD FDSRCPS
Senior Lecturer, Prosthetic Dentistry, School of Dentistry,
The University of Birmingham, UK

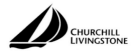

**CHURCHILL LIVINGSTONE**

EDINBURGH LONDON MADRID MELBOURNE NEW YORK SAN FRANCISCO
TOKYO 1998

CHURCHILL LIVINGSTONE
Medical Division of Pearson Professional Limited

Distributed in the United States of America by
Churchill Livingstone Inc., 650 Avenue of the
Americas, New York, N.Y. 10011, and by
associated companies, branches and
representatives throughout the world.

© Pearson Professional Limited 1998

Second Edition 1998

ISBN 0443 05813 X

**British Library Cataloguing in Publication Data**
A catalogue record for this book is available from
the British Library.

**Library of Congress Cataloging in Publication Data**
A catalog record for this book is available from
the Library of Congress.

Medical knowledge is constantly
changing. As new information
becomes available, changes in
treatment, procedures, equipment
and the use of drugs become
necessary. The authors and the
publishers have, as far as it is
possible, taken care to ensure
that the information given in this
text is accurate and up to date.
However, readers are strongly
advised to confirm that the
information, especially with
regard to drug usage, complies
with current legislation and
standards of practice.

The
publisher's
policy is to use
**paper manufactured
from sustainable forests**

*For Churchill Livingstone*

*Publisher:* Michael Parkinson
*Project manager:* Ninette Premdas
*Project editor:* Jim Killgore
*Design:* Erik Bigland
*Project controller:* Kay Hunston

Prduced by Longmern Asia Limited, Hong Kong.
SWTC/01

# Preface

This book is intended to be a revision aid in the field of restorative dentistry. Various procedures and techniques involved in the speciality of restorative dentistry are shown. Indications and contraindications for the different treatment modalities are discussed. The text and illustrations are not meant to be extensive but serve as a starting point which will stimulate the reader to follow up an interest in this subject area.

The authors would like to acknowledge the support and assistance of Professor W. R. E. Laird, head of the teaching unit of Prosthetic Dentistry at the University of Birmingham, in the production of this book.

Birmingham
1998

C.W.B.
A.D.W.

# Foreword

With the academic and technical advances which are occurring in dentistry, it is inevitable that this must be accompanied by increases in the educational and descriptive texts available in the form of new books.

Dentistry, however, is essentially a relatively limited profession, and when one considers the international variation in clinical and technical skills coupled with perceived need for dental care and the funding available, any new textbook must be able to present in a clear manner advances which are to the benefit of society. In particular, care must be taken to avoid repetition whilst attempting to cover the subject adequately.

This has been achieved well by the authors in their first text, which serves to bring together the concepts of removable and fixed prosthodontics in a single volume, and is particularly appropriate in the current climate in the United Kingdom of General Professional Training and Specialisation. The choice of a colour atlas with a limited amount of text is an unsurpassed way to present updates in knowledge and technique to the busy practitioner in a manner which is easily understood, not only by the clinician but also the technician and most importantly, the patient. The authors are to be congratulated for identifying a gap in the market and for filling it so effectively. This book will be of benefit to all practitioners in Restorative Dentistry.

1998
Professor W.R.E. Laird

Professor of Dental Prosthetics/Honorary Consultant in Restorative Dentistry, University of Birmingham, UK

# Contents

## Squamous cell carcinoma

*Aetiology and pathology*

The aetiology of squamous cell carcinoma (Fig. 1) is unclear, although there appears to be a higher incidence amongst heavy smokers and drinkers. Certain intraoral conditions are also described as being premalignant in nature; these include lichen planus, dysplastic leukoplakia, candidosis, submucous fibrosis.

*Diagnosis*

Differentiation by clinical examination of the lesion (Fig. 2) from more common clinical lesions such as an area of hyperplasia is often possible. However, histological examination of the region (Fig. 3) is always required to confirm the diagnosis.

*Management*

Surgical excision, radiotherapy and chemotherapy can all be used in the treatment of oral carcinoma. However, most oral cancers respond poorly to chemotherapy leaving surgical excision and the use of adjunctive radiotherapy as the more common treatments of choice. There appears to be an increase in the incidence of oral carcinoma, although a widespread geographical variance in incidence is evident, with it being more common on the Indian subcontinent.

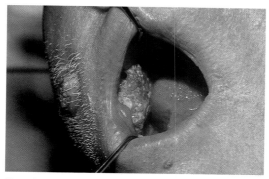

**Fig. 1** Squamous cell carcinoma in cheek.

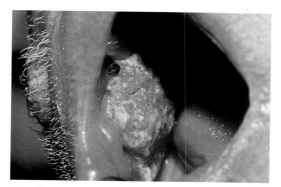

**Fig. 2** Close up of lesion.

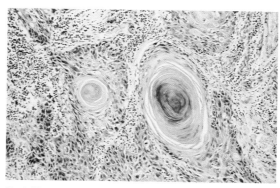

**Fig. 3** Microscopic appearance of the squamous cell carcinoma.

# Denture-induced hyperplasia

*Aetiology and pathology*

Denture-induced hyperplasia is caused by trauma from an overextended denture periphery or an unretentive, unstable denture base. It is seen more frequently in the lower arch rather than the upper (Figs 4 & 5) and is often related to poorly controlled follow-up of an immediate denture.

*Diagnosis*

Denture-induced hyperplasia presents as single or multiple flaps of fibrous tissue related to the border of a denture base (Fig. 6).

*Management*

Removal of the offending denture allows for complete resolution in respect of small lesions. It may also be possible to trim the border of the denture and apply a tissue conditioning material to improve stability and retention. This will result in less trauma to the site. If the hyperplastic lesion is large, however, it is often necessary to undertake surgical removal of the tissue. In any event the denture must always be discarded for 2–3 weeks prior to surgery to allow as much natural resolution as possible. Chronic irritation is a possible cause of oral carcinoma and therefore all hyperplastic tissue should be examined histologically to discount this.

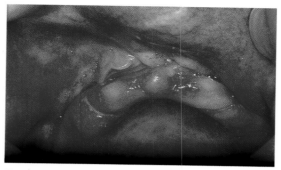

**Fig. 4** Denture hyperplasia of upper ridge.

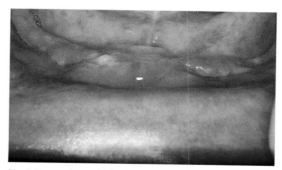

**Fig. 5** Denture hyperplasia of lower ridge.

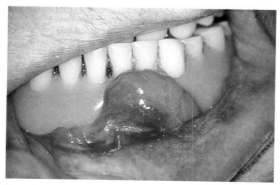

**Fig. 6** Causative denture in place.

# Assorted soft tissue disorders

**Pregnancy epulis** (Fig. 7)

*Aetiology and pathology*

Subgingival calculus or an overhanging restoration can be the simple cause of this exaggerated inflammatory lesion of the attached mucosa.

*Diagnosis*

A female patient with a localised gingival swelling who confirms she is pregnant. On histological examination the tissue is extremely vascular and is heavily infiltrated with polymorphs.

*Management*

Improvement of the patient's oral hygiene, sometimes combined with surgical excision of the lesion. If left untreated this condition resolves spontaneously after birth.

**Fibroepithelial polyp** (Fig. 8)

*Aetiology and pathology*

Chronic trauma from cheek biting resulting in fibrous hyperplasia.

*Diagnosis*

Differentiate from other possible soft tissue lesions by histological examination of the excised lesion.

*Management*

Excisional removal and histological confirmation.

**Wegener's granulomatosis** (Fig. 9)

*Aetiology and pathology*

This disease is thought to be an immune-complex disorder.

*Diagnosis*

The characteristic form of 'strawberry' gingivitis can be pathognomic. However confirmation by histological examination will confirm this diagnosis with a picture of necrotising vasculitis and characteristic giant cells.

*Management*

Chemotherapy or co-trimoxazole are the treatments of choice.

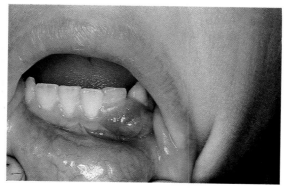

**Fig. 7** Pregnancy epulis.

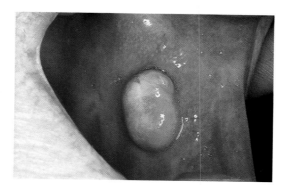

**Fig. 8** Fibroepithelial polyp.

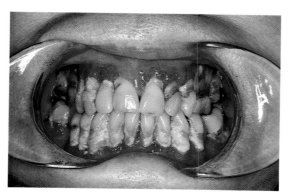

**Fig. 9** Wegener's granulomatosis.

# Denture-induced stomatitis

*Aetiology and pathology*

This is a multifactorial condition, the factors predisposing to which include: poor denture hygiene, trauma from an ill-fitting denture base, *candida albicans*, endocrine imbalance, iron deficiency anaemia, reduced salivary flow, folate deficiency, and diabetes mellitus. It has been shown that this condition affects women more frequently than men.

*Diagnosis*

The clinical picture is classically a diffuse erythema associated purely with the denture bearing area (Figs 10 & 11). It is most commonly asymptomatic and therefore the synonym denture sore mouth should be discarded.

*Management*

Establishing and controlling possible general aetiological factors (Fig. 12):
- Correct oral and denture hygiene. Dentures should be soaked in a hypochlorite solution.
- Correction of the ill-fitting nature of the dentures.
- Use of antifungals such as amphotericin, miconazole and nystatin.
- Removing the dentures at night.

If these simple measures do not resolve the problem, haemotological investigations will be required.

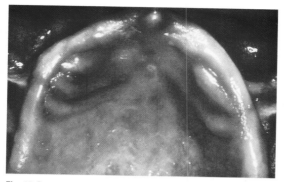

**Fig. 10** Denture stomatitis—upper arch of a complete denture patient.

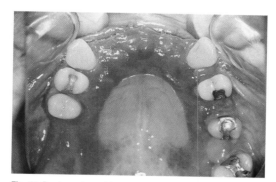

**Fig. 11** Denture stomatitis—upper arch under a cobalt/chromium partial denture.

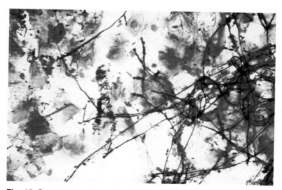

**Fig. 12** Smear taken from the denture surface of a patient showing fungal hyphae.

## Cotton wool burn

*Aetiology and pathology*

Oral tissues may suffer localised dryness during isolation and aspiration procedures. If a dry cotton wool roll is present and removed from the sulcus it may adhere to the tissues, removing the superficial thin friable layer of the lining mucosa (Figs 13 & 14).

*Diagnosis*

The classic clinical appearance is of a large sloughed ulcer in the buccal sulcus adjacent to a recently restored tooth. Other factors which could have resulted in a similar appearance include incorrect isolation or removal of acid etch gel or dentine conditioners.

*Management*

Reassurance that the area will heal unscarred. The patient should be discouraged from the use of any proprietary gel formulations which, although relieving the pain, often just *burn* the region (Fig. 15) resulting in later discomfort. This area will heal in a few days and if required the use of topical anaesthetic agents may ease the discomfort during this period.

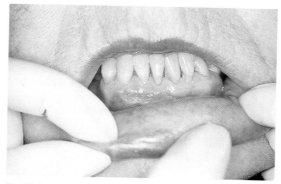

**Fig. 13** Cotton wool burn—lower lip.

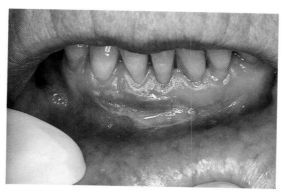

**Fig. 14** Cotton wool burn—labial sulcus.

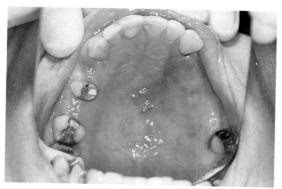

**Fig. 15** Bonjela burn.

# Leukaemia

*Aetiology and
pathology*

Leukaemia is idiopathic in origin although various attempts have been made to link it to radiation. Leukaemia represents a malignant proliferation of white cells, replacing their normal development in the bone marrow. This process may affect any of the white cell strains but most commonly occurs in the lymphocytes, monocytes or granulocytes. Leukaemia may exist in either acute or chronic forms (Figs 16, 17 & 18).

*Diagnosis*

In acute forms of this disease, it is common for oral symptoms to develop first. These can include: oral bleeding, petechiae, ulceration, mucosal pallor, oral infections—candidosis or herpetic; and extraorally cervical lymphadenopathy. Confirmation of the clinical diagnosis involves haematological analysis and bone marrow biopsy.

*Management*

Management of these patients is dependent on which type of leukaemia is present. Commonly potent cytotoxic drugs are used or sometimes radiotherapy. In some types destruction of all white cells and marrow, followed by a bone marrow transplant is required. It is important therefore that these patients carry out a strict oral hygiene regime to minimise the risk of infection from the oral environment.

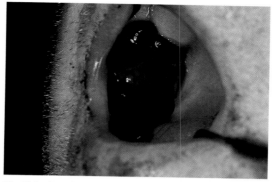

**Fig. 16** Leukaemia—appearance of right cheek.

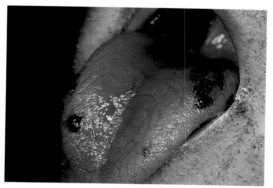

**Fig. 17** Leukaemia—appearance of tongue.

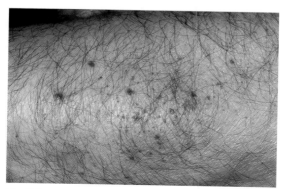

**Fig. 18** Leukaemia—appearance of forearm.

## Keratocyst

*Aetiology and pathology*

The cyst is thought to arise from the epithelium of the tooth primordium (dental lamina) or its residues (Figs 19, 20 & 21).

*Diagnosis*

The odontogenic keratocyst has a characteristic though not pathognomic, radiological appearance. Of keratocysts 70% appear in the mandible, normally at the mandibular angle and ascending ramus. The radiographic appearance is normally of a multilobular lesion, which causes expansion of the cortical bone. Aspiration biopsy may be possible and identification of epithelial squames from this is diagnostic. However such a sample cannot always be obtained and often an incisional biopsy and histological examination is required to confirm the diagnosis.

*Management*

The reported frequency of recurrence of these lesions is reputed to be due to incomplete removal of the cyst lining in one piece. There is conflicting evidence that recurrence is related to the surgical treatment of this lesion. Enucleation is the surgical treatment of choice although size and position may dictate the use of a marsupialisation technique. Enucleation combined with the removal of the overlying mucoperiostium may further reduce the risk of recurrence. The most important features affecting the recurrence rate appear to be the size and location of the lesion.

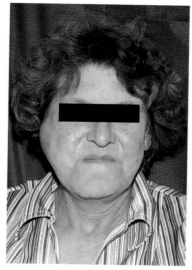

**Fig. 19** Keratocyst—extraoral.

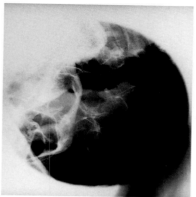

**Fig. 20** Keratocyst—external oblique view.

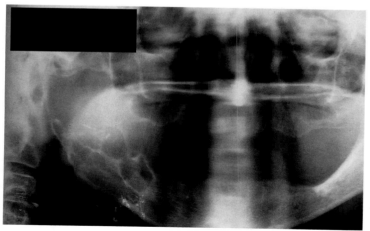

**Fig. 21** Keratocyst—panoramic view.

## Torus palatinus and torus mandibularis

*Aetiology and pathology*

Genetic in origin and more commonly seen in women than men, they are bony, commonly asymptomatic and slow growing.

*Diagnosis*

- Palatal tori (Figs 22 & 23) appear in the midline of the palate and neoplasia should be excluded from the diagnosis.
- Mandibular tori (Fig. 24) are bilateral, elevated and lingual to the mandibular premolars. Unerupted teeth should be discounted in this situation.

*Management*

These hard tissue excrescences require no management as such but often pose problems if dentures are to be constructed in the region. Palatal relief over the palatine torus will help prevent repeated fracture of the denture base, and careful extension of the lingual flanges in the mandibular tori region can avoid any potential problems.

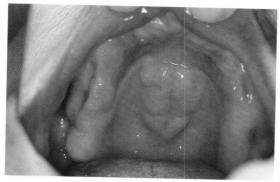

**Fig. 22** Palatine torus.

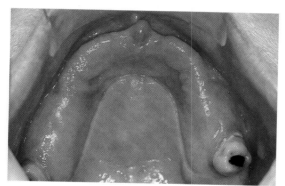

**Fig. 23** Palatine torus.

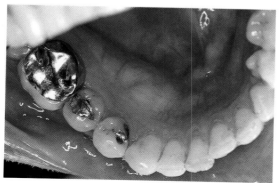

**Fig. 24** Mandibular torus.

## Severe resorption

*Aetiology and pathology*

Residual ridge resorption occurs in the mandible and maxilla after removal of the natural teeth and might be considered as a form of disuse atrophy. The resorptive process occurs at different rates in the maxilla and mandible such that the mandible commonly resorbs at a rate of 4 : 1 to that of the maxilla. This process will continue indefinitely and can be affected by various factors including hormone levels, smoking and some as yet unidentified factors.

*Diagnosis*

When severe resorption occurs, the mandible in particular becomes very thin and all that may remain is its lower border (Figs 25, 26 & 27). In such circumstances the mandible is described as being pipe-stemmed and the inferior alveolar nerve comes to lie on its superior surface. This can present the patient and clinician with several problems including possible physiological fracture of the severely weakened bone or pain from pressure on the nerve which is now placed superficially.

*Management*

The placement of implants into the edentulous ridges or maintenance of roots as overdenture abutments has been shown to preserve bone and prevent this severe bony resorption occurring. Attempts to apply bone grafts using autogenous as well as artificial bone, and the use of barrier membrane materials have all been tried in an attempt to augment resorbed ridges.

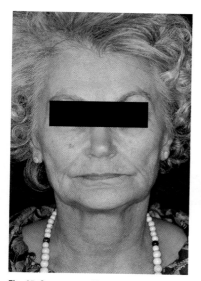

**Fig. 25** Severe mandibular atrophy—extraoral.

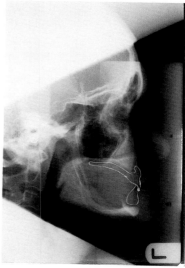

**Fig. 26** Severe mandibular atrophy—lateral cephalometric view.

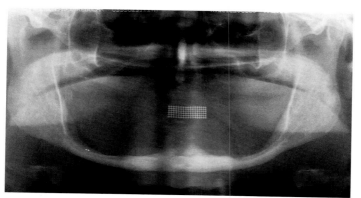

**Fig. 27** Severe mandibular atrophy—panoramic view.

## Clinical appearance of severe mandibular resorption

*Aetiology and pathology*

Bone resorption occurs in the mandible at a faster rate than the maxilla and therefore the presentation of a severely atrophic mandible in a patient who has been edentulous for a considerable period is not uncommon. The aetiological factors for this process have been outlined previously.

*Diagnosis*

The clinical appearance of an atrophic mandible (Figs 28 & 29) is the loss of height and width together with relative loss of the depth of the buccal and lingual sulci. There is an accompanying loss of attached mucosa overlying this situation. This has important implications for the placement of a satisfactory prosthesis as the retention and stability will be affected by the ridge form and the area available for support will also be reduced.

*Management*

The relative superficial nature of the attaching muscles to the mandible such as the buccinator, mylohyoid and genioglossus is a direct result of the loss of bony height. The genial tubercles (Fig. 30) also become higher in relative terms to the residual ridge and this may compromise the placement of any prosthesis.

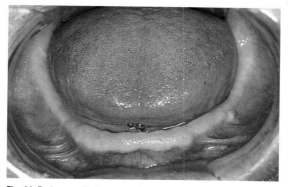

**Fig. 28** Early mandibular resorption.

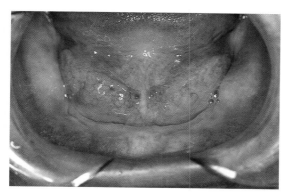

**Fig. 29** Mandibular resorption.

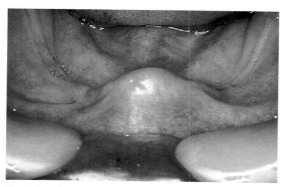

**Fig. 30** Prominent genial tubercles.

## Periodontal disease/root caries

*Aetiology and pathology*

Dental bacterial plaque is the major aetiological factor in both these hard tissue disorders. In periodontal disease it has been demonstrated that organisms present in microbial plaque, or substances derived from them, constitute the primary aetiological agent in inflammatory gingival and periodontal diseases. Some plaque bacteria ferment dietary carbohydrate producing acids that—acting in susceptible dental sites, particularly root surfaces—result in carious lesions.

*Diagnosis*

*Periodontal breakdown* (Fig. 31) can be assessed clinically by the use of loss of attachment charting used in conjunction with clinical radiographs (Fig. 32).

*Root caries* can be detected by careful examination using a dry field and good illumination of the region (Fig. 33). Confirmation of the lesion can be gained by either bite-wing or periapical radiographs of the tooth involved.

*Management*

Prevention in both cases is the best form of management. This would involve good oral hygiene measures to prevent plaque accumulation and dietary advice to reduce the amount of fermentable carbohydrate available.

Clearly intervention will be required when the disease process has progressed and therefore conservative treatment and periodontal management will no longer just involve preventative measures.

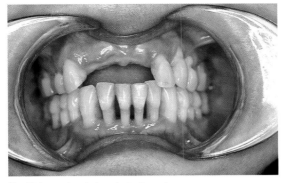

**Fig. 31** Loss of periodontal attachment.

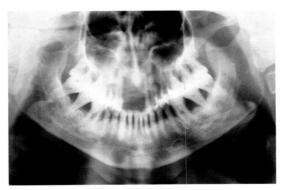

**Fig. 32** Radiographic appearance of periodontal bone loss.

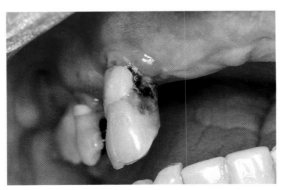

**Fig. 33** Root caries.

# Periodontal acrylic veneer

*Definition*

A facing that is placed buccal to the natural dentition and constructed in acrylic resin. It masks any recession or postsurgical tissue loss that is present (Figs 34 & 35) and gives the appearance of a normal gingival contour and level.

*Management*

Such a prosthesis (Fig. 36) should only be constructed for a patient whose oral hygiene is good and whose periodontal condition is controlled. Veneers utilise both the interproximal area of the dental arch together with salivary adhesion for their retention. They should not be worn when sleeping on both periodontal health and medico-legal grounds.

*Advantages*

- The major advantage of this appliance is the improvement in appearance that can be achieved particularly in a patient who has a high lip line.
- This veneer can also have the beneficial action of improving speech, as often patients who suffer from marked anterior recession feel that a 'whistling' problem can result during speech due to the development of large interproximal spaces. If these are filled by such an appliance, the problem is normally resolved.

*Disadvantages*

Like most prostheses there is the potential for increased plaque accumulation if the patient does not maintain a high level of oral hygiene.

*Procedure*

A special impression tray which supports a buccal impression is used. The impression is taken from a buccal path of insertion/withdrawal and modern elastomers can cope effectively with the undercut areas.

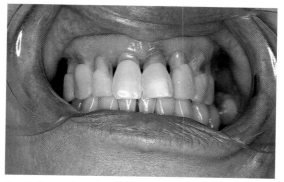

Fig. 34 Severe gingival recession.

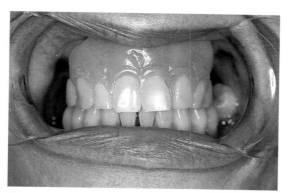

Fig. 35 Periodontal acrylic veneer masking recession.

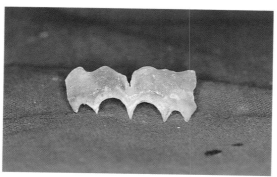

Fig. 36 Periodontal acrylic veneer out of the mouth.

# Root resection

*Definition*

A procedure where one or two roots of a multirooted tooth are amputated, leaving the crown to be supported by the remaining root or roots (Figs 37, 38 & 39).

*Indications*

- Single roots of a multirooted tooth that cannot be treated by conventional root canal therapy or retrograde techniques because of lateral canals, calcification, dilaceration, pulp stones, perforations, broken instruments or loss of bony support for that individual root.
- Multirooted teeth with individual root fractures.
- Severe vertical bone loss affecting one root of a multirooted tooth.
- Inadequate maintenance of a furcation lesion because of access problems.

*Management*

The most important factor in relation to a tooth which has had a root resected is that the root is severed as close to the furcation as possible. This allows for better patient access to the region together with an enhanced gingival contour, resulting in improved gingival health of the site.

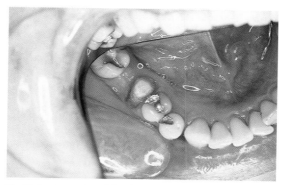

**Fig. 37** Root resection of distal root of a mandibular first molar.

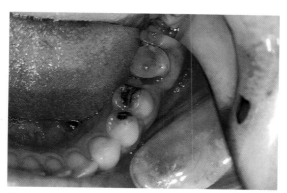

**Fig. 38** Root resection of mesial root of a mandibular first molar.

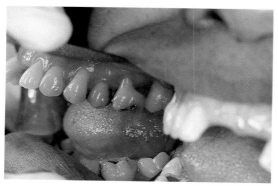

**Fig. 39** Root resection of distobuccal root of a maxillary first molar.

## Tetracycline staining

*Aetiology and pathology*

Tetracycline staining is a cause of tooth discoloration which occurs when these broad spectrum antiobiotics are given to pregnant women or children under the age of 12 (as crown calcification of molars has not been completed before this).

*Diagnosis*

The clinical appearance is of yellow, brown or greyish hyperpigmentation of the affected dentition (Figs 40, 41 & 42). The teeth affected may also be hypoplastic. Together with a relevant history this should provide a clear clinical diagnosis and should not be confused with amelogenesis imperfecta, dentinogenesis imperfecta or fluorosis.

*Management*

Bleaching can be attempted for mild forms of this condition. As the staining is intrinsic, however, this only works in a relatively small number of cases. The more common treatment is the placement of porcelain veneers or, for extremely severe cases, full veneer crowns.

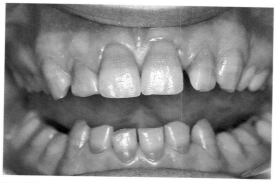

**Fig. 40** Severe tetracycline staining.

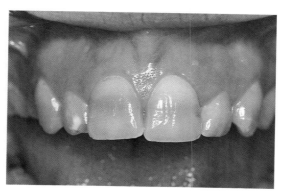

**Fig. 41** Tetracycline staining.

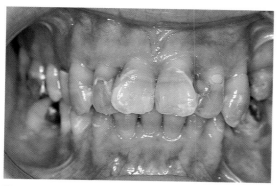

**Fig. 42** Tetracycline staining aesthetically exacerbated by gingival recession.

# Amelogenesis imperfecta

*Aetiology and pathology*

Genetic in origin with a wide variety of presentations (Figs 43, 44 & 45).

*Diagnosis*

There are three main types:

*Hypocalcified.* Although the enamel matrix is normal there has been inadequate calcification. The enamel is often opaque and may exhibit a wide variety of discolorations. It is soft and easily lost.

*Hypoplastic.* Although the calcification is normal the enamel matrix is defective. The enamel therefore is hard and shiny but malformed. It may be prone to staining.

*Hypomaturation* is described as giving a snow-capped appearance, where the underlying enamel has not matured fully but may have a thin layer of mature enamel overlying it.

Differentation should be made from other causes of tooth discoloration.

*Management*

The management of such cases can be part of a complex restorative treatment plan depending upon the severity of the condition. Restorative intervention may be required to protect the underlying tooth structure because of the poor enamel quality. Treatment may be needed for purely aesthetic reasons.

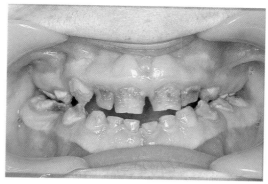

**Fig. 43** Amelogenesis imperfecta.

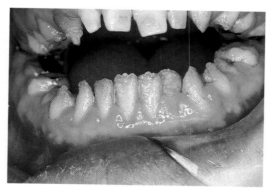

**Fig. 44** Amelogenesis imperfecta.

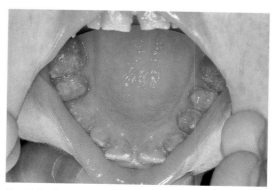

**Fig. 45** Amelogenesis imperfecta.

## Normal anatomy

### Upper denture bearing area

This includes the hard palate together with the functional sulcus. The posterior extent of the upper denture bearing area is at the junction of hard and soft palate. In Figure 46 the ridges are well formed and the palatogingival vestige may be seen. This, together with the incisive papilla, is used as a biometric guideline for the positioning of upper artificial teeth. The underlying support may be firm if there is sufficient bone present. An unsupported ridge will consist of a greater amount of fibrous tissue due to localised bone resorption without associated reduction in soft tissue. The palatal area provides good support and is relatively resistant to resorption.

### Lower denture bearing area (Figs 47 & 48)

This includes the supporting ridges and extends to the functional sulcus. The area of support is reduced by the presence of the tongue and the posterior extent is half way up the retromolar pad. Support may be gained from the buccal shelf of bone which is present buccally to the posterior aspect of the residual ridge. In cases of severe mandibular resorption muscle attachments such as the genioglossus and the mylohyoid will become more prominent and may produce problems with soreness under the denture during function.

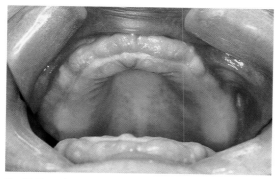

**Fig. 46** Normal anatomy—upper edentulous arch.

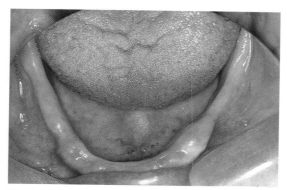

**Fig. 47** Normal anatomy—lower edentulous arch.

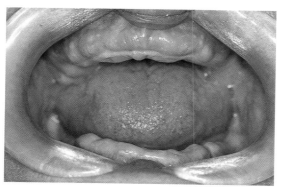

**Fig. 48** Normal anatomy—anterior view of arches.

# Impression materials

Several impression materials are used for complete denture construction. These include: impression compound, impression plaster, low and high viscosity alginate, zinc oxide and eugenol paste, low and medium viscosity elastomers (Figs 49, 50 & 51).

An impression material may have either mucodisplacive or mucostatic properties.

- A mucodisplacive material is of high viscosity and will displace the underlying soft tissues similar to loading under function.
- A mucostatic material is of low viscosity and will result in minimal distortion of the tissues during impression taking and this may be used to optimise retention of the denture.

Each impression material will have different properties as outlined in the table below:

| Material | Property | Elastic | Accuracy | Stability |
|---|---|---|---|---|
| Impression compound | Mucodisplacive | No | Poor | Poor |
| Impression plaster | Mucostatic | No | Good | Good |
| Low viscosity alginate | Mucostatic | Yes | Good | Poor |
| High viscosity alginate | Mucodisplacive | Yes | Good | Poor |
| Zinc oxide and eugenol | Mucostatic | No | Good | Good |
| Low and medium viscosity elastomeric materials | Mucostatic | Yes | Good | Good |

The choice of material will depend on the clinical situation and the clinical need. For instance a poorly fitting stock tray will benefit from the use of impression compound as it will support itself and make good the deficiencies of the tray. Alginate is an accurate material but is not dimensionally stable with time. Elastomeric materials are relatively expensive compared to the other materials and are used where there are large undercuts present.

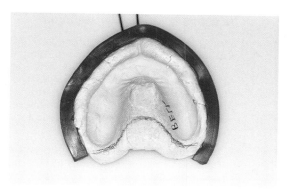

**Fig. 49** Impression materials—plaster of Paris.

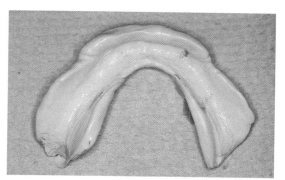

**Fig. 50** Impression materials—zinc oxide/eugenol.

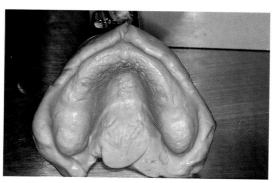

**Fig. 51** Impression materials—alginate.

# Selective compression technique

This is based on the assumption that, in the presence of an unsupported ridge, the patient has a problem of support or stability of the denture rather than retention during function. The technique aims therefore to apply controlled loading to the tissues in order to stabilise them against the underlying bone and also to dissipate the load.

1. An impression should first be obtained in a mucostatic material (plaster) to record the tissues under minimal load. This is recorded in a stock tray and the resultant cast can be considered as an accurate reproduction of the denture bearing area.
2. An impression is now recorded of the **master cast** in impression compound used in thin section (Fig. 52).
3. The surface of the impression is flamed and re-adapted to the cast.
4. The impression is placed in the mouth. It should be stable and retentive.
5. The area of unsupported tissue in the mouth (Fig. 53) is outlined on the impression.
6. The rest of the impression is lightly flamed and inserted into the mouth under load.
7. This will now be the master impression. On the cast poured from this, a heat cured permanent base should be constructed for the registration and trial.

**NB** It is unnecessary to take a wash impression in the compound, which may defeat the object of the exercise.

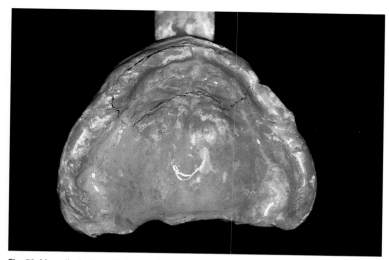

**Fig. 52** Mucodisplacive with impression compound.

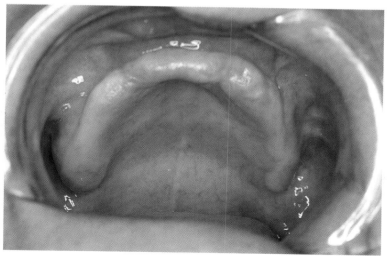

**Fig. 53** Anterior flabby ridge.

# Mucostatic impression technique

*Aim*

This is based on the assumption that, in the presence of an unsupported ridge (Fig. 54), the patient has a problem of retention of the denture during rest. The technique aims to apply mucosal loading to the supporting tissue and take a mucostatic impression of the unsupported ridge.

*Procedure*

1. An impression should first be obtained in a mucostatic material (i.e. plaster or low viscosity alginate) to record the tissues under minimal load. This is recorded in stock tray and the resultant cast can be considered as an accurate reproduction of the denture bearing area.
2. An individual closely adapted tray is constructed with a window cut over the unsupported region. As a result of this the handle has to be placed in the midline of the palate.
3. The tray is checked for extension in the mouth and the periphery is border moulded as required with autopolymerising acrylic resin.
4. A zinc oxide and eugenol paste impression is then taken of the ridge (Fig. 55). Once this is set the impression is removed and the excess material which has flowed into the window region is cut away using a scalpel.
5. The impression is then reseated in the patient's mouth and a fluid mix of plaster applied to the unsupported ridge area. To ensure a good junction between the zinc oxide and eugenol paste and plaster the three-in-one syringe is employed to manipulate the plaster.
6. Once set the impression is removed and checked for accuracy and then sent to the laboratory for casting.

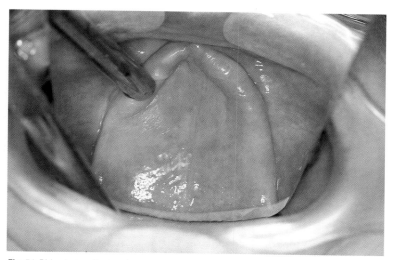

**Fig. 54** Ridge being displaced.

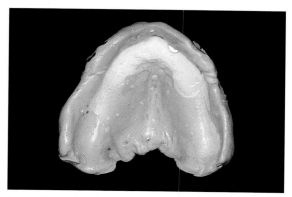

**Fig. 55** Mucostatic using ZOE and Plaster of Paris.

# Conventional complete dentures

*Definition*

A conventional complete denture is one made by taking impressions of the upper and lower denture bearing areas; it is constructed using identifiable anatomical structures and relationships.

*Indications*

The replacement of natural teeth by a removable prosthesis may require that the clinician makes changes in the overall construction which are greater than those that can be accommodated by copying the patient's previous dentures. In some cases there may be no previous dentures present and construction of new dentures would follow the stages outlined above.

*Advantages*

The clinician has control of the changes that are required. There is an opportunity to undertake impressions of the denture bearing tissues under optimal conditions. Changes in the jaw relationship together with muscle support may be modified and assessed using ideal parameters.

*Disadvantages*

Adaptability to large changes brought about during conventional denture construction may be poor. Copy dentures for instance have an advantage in that the polished surfaces are often in an ideal position relative to the soft tissues of the cheeks, lips and tongue. Using a conventional technique the ideal positioning of the polished surfaces may not be immediately apparent until the patient has worn the dentures.

*Procedure*

A conventional complete denture is constructed in the following sequence:
1. Preliminary impressions in stock trays followed by master impressions in an individual tray constructed on the preliminary cast.
2. Registration of the jaw relationship (Fig. 56).
3. Trial dentures constructed in wax (Fig. 57).
4. Insertion or placement of the finished dentures (Fig. 58).
5. Review of any problems during wearing of the dentures.

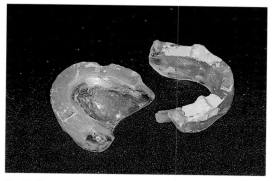

**Fig. 56** Upper and lower wax rims sealed with bite registration paste and then separated.

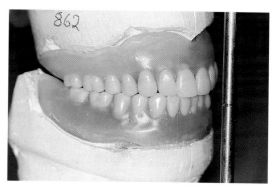

**Fig. 57** Complete dentures at wax try-in stage.

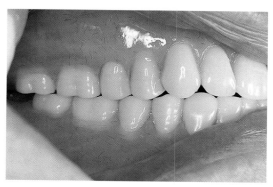

**Fig. 58** Complete dentures inserted and the occlusion being refined.

# Aesthetics of complete dentures

*Definition*

The appearance of complete dentures should follow similar principles to that of the natural dentition.

*Procedure*

Aesthetics of a prosthesis depend upon the colour, shape and size of the artificial teeth, their orientation relative to each other and the arch form (Fig. 59). The colour of a tooth should be influenced by several features, which include the age of the patient, the race and complexion of the patient and the patient's preference. Shape and size of a tooth should reflect the sex, age and personality of the patient but most importantly their facial and overall contour.

The orientation or spacing of each tooth in relation to its neighbours can have a profound influence on the overall appearance of the finished denture (Figs 60 & 61). If the patient had a diastema between the upper central incisors in the natural dentition, the placement of such a feature in the new prosthesis will reduce the often unwanted change that can occur in the appearance of a patient with a new prosthesis. If possible a complete denture should follow the arch form and occlusal plane of the previous natural dentition. This is most readily achieved if an immediate denture has been constructed for the patient. This denture will possess all the original features of the patient's natural dentition which will then be reproduced in the new prosthesis.

Many other techniques such as tinting, colouring and contouring the gingiva on the denture base can affect the final appearance created by a denture.

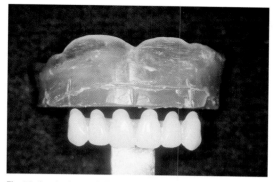

**Fig. 59** Aesthetics—relationship of anterior teeth to upper occlusal rim.

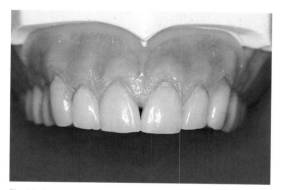

**Fig. 60** Arrangement of irregular teeth.

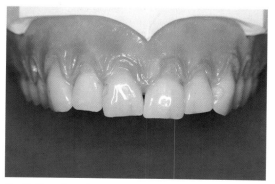

**Fig. 61** Gross irregularity of artificial teeth.

## Techniques

*Definition*

A copy denture preserves the polished surface of the existing prosthesis while allowing modifications to be carried out to the fitting and occlusal surfaces of a complete denture. As a patient's adaptive potential decreases with age the maintenance of the shape of the original polished surface results in less adjustment of the supporting musculature being required. Therefore the title 'Copy denture technique' is really a misnomer as it is only rarely that an exact copy of an existing denture will be required.

*Indications*

- An elderly patient presenting with upper and lower complete dentures which have been satisfactory for many years but are now loose or worn.
- A patient with a history of denture problems where it may be useful to make controlled modifications in the copy denture of the most successful previous dentures.
- Previous immediate dentures which require replacing after bone resorption following extractions.
- Second 'spare' set of dentures.

*Advantages*

- No alteration or mutilation of existing denture (as occurs in a reline or rebase).
- No period for patient to be without dentures (as occurs in a reline or rebase).
- Reduced number of clinical stages.
- Simple duplication procedure.

*Disadvantages*

- Technical support for such techniques is variable.
- Various clinical techniques are available (Figs 62, 63 & 64) (Laboratories may prefer only one method).
- Laboratory charges can be variable.

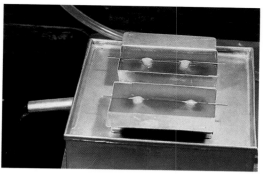

**Fig. 62** Use of reversible hydrocolloid to copy dentures.

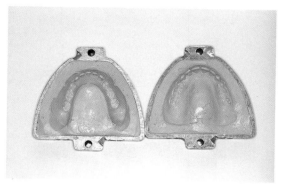

**Fig. 63** Murray/Woolland technique.

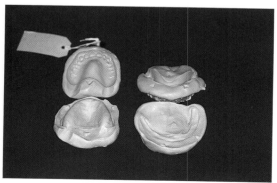

**Fig. 64** Replica record block technique.

## Standard copy technique

*Definition*

As previously described.

*Indications*

As previously described.

*Advantages*

- The reproduction of successful design features on which a patient's tolerance and control of the previous dentures depend.
- The accurate alteration of undesirable features.
- Simplified occlusal registration and a reduced number of clinical visits.

*Disadvantages*

Increased charges may be made by commercial laboratories. The production of a template and the need for the technician to follow this exactly also often makes this technique unpopular amongst technical staff.

*Procedure*

1. A mould of the original denture that is being copied is produced by whichever method the clinician wishes to use (Fig. 65). This is poured up, with the teeth in wax and the bases in self-cured acrylic. A stone duplicate is also poured as a guide to the original denture, both in respect of the polished surfaces and tooth position.
2. The wax and acrylic copy denture is then either used as a registration block or, if minimal occlusal alteration is required, taken to the trial stage (Fig. 66 & 67).
3. The dentures are tried in and the occlusion and vertical dimension checked. If this is found to be satisfactory any undercuts are removed from the baseplates and a wash impression is taken within both the upper and lower bases using a closed mouth technique.
4. A master cast is then poured and the finished dentures processed in the normal manner.

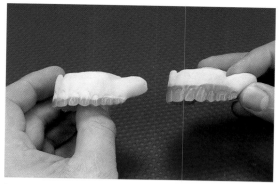

**Fig. 65** Standard copy denture technique—template.

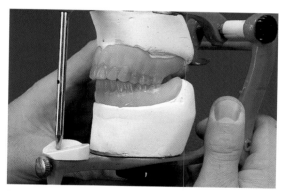

**Fig. 66** Templates placed on average movement articulator.

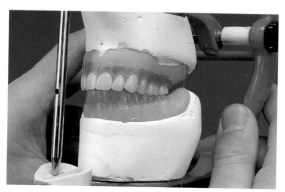

**Fig. 67** Set-up of copy denture templates.

## Copy denture for severe tooth wear

*Definition*

A duplicate denture made with as few modifications to the previous existing denture as possible.

*Indications*

Patients who present with mutilated dentures (Fig. 68) that they can comfortably wear and who have a history of intolerance to conventional replacement of these dentures. Clinically, there may be a place for providing the patient with a copy of their old dentures with as few modifications as possible (Figs 69 & 70). This will improve the chances of patient acceptance of the new prosthesis.

*Advantages*

It is likely that the patient's acceptance of and adaptation to such a denture will be high as it will not be different to their 'tried and trusted' set. A further advantage is the reduction in numerous remakes.

*Disadvantages*

By following such a technique, the clinician may unknowingly copy faults that may in the long term cause such problems as TMJ symptoms and denture instability.

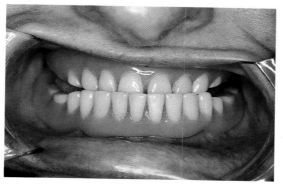

**Fig. 68** Severe tooth wear copy denture—presentation.

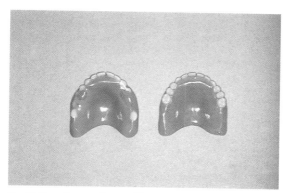

**Fig. 69** Copy denture after modification with original dentures.

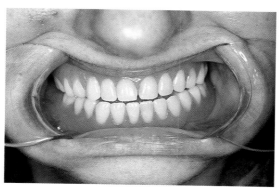

**Fig. 70** Final clinical result.

## Complete upper overdenture

*Definition*

A prosthesis that derives its support and sometimes retention from one or more abutment teeth which may have been reduced in height (Figs 71 & 72).

*Management*

The retention of roots of natural teeth provides improved stability to a denture as well a maintaining alveolar bone. Roots should be used as overdenture abutments when the standard of oral hygiene is high and there is good periodontal support.

*Advantages*

The alveolar bone is retained around these teeth and also between them. By keeping the teeth, the proprioceptive fibres of the periodontal membrane help in maintaining sensory feedback and allow more rapid adaptation to the dentures.

*Disadvantages*

Overdentures may require advanced conservative techniques such as endodontics and occasionally gold copings. Such procedures may increase the cost of the treatment.

*Procedure*

The abutment teeth require to be reduced in height to 1–2 mm above the gingival margin. The coronal shape produced is preferably dome-shaped. The construction of the removable prosthesis continues along traditional treatment lines and the overdenture encloses the reduced teeth (Fig. 73).

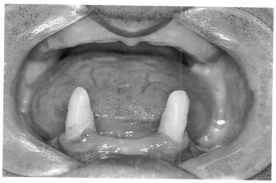

**Fig. 71** Classic presentation of a case suitable for overdentures.

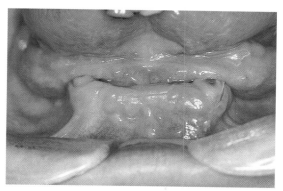

**Fig. 72** Reduction of teeth following root canal therapy.

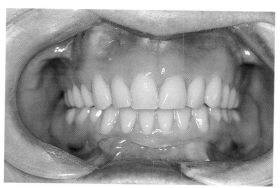

**Fig. 73** Overdentures in place.

## Tooth wear overdenture

*Definition*

A removable tooth-borne overdenture which is used to restore a dentition that has undergone severe tooth loss. There is some degree of overlap between onlay and overdentures in the management of such a problem.

*Indications*

The overdenture option may be used if there has been extensive loss of tooth substance (Fig. 74) and its replacement is not possible using fixed restorations.

*Advantages*

This option can quickly restore function and aesthetics. It is reversible if there are problems with patient adaptation.

*Disadvantages*

There is extensive coverage of the dentition by the removable prosthesis. This may increase the incidence of periodontal problems and caries attack. Cost may increase if there is a need for a cast cobalt/chromium baseplate.

*Procedure*

1. Such clinical procedures will require treatment planning on casts mounted on an articulator.
2. The construction of the overdentures may require tooth preparation prior to impression taking if there is inadequate occlusal clearance for the denture base or if the coronal margins are sharp or unsupported.
3. See Figures 75 and 76.

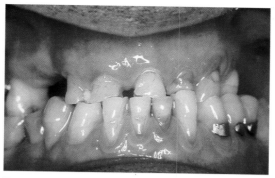

**Fig. 74** Initial presentation of a tooth wear case.

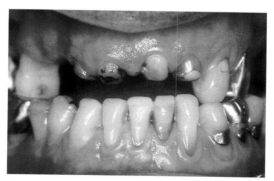

**Fig. 75** The reduction of the overdenture abutments.

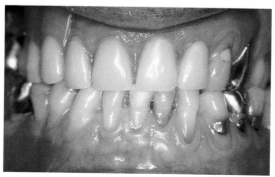

**Fig. 76** Final overdenture in place. (Courtesy of Mrs E.A. McLaughlin)

# 6 / Immediate replacement dentures

*Definition* | A denture that is made prior to the extraction of the natural teeth and which is inserted into the mouth immediately after the extraction of those teeth.

*Indications* | Patients may require extraction of teeth due to caries or periodontal disease or for aesthetic reasons (Fig. 77).

*Advantages* | Original appearance is maintained by placing the artificial teeth in a position similar to natural teeth or improved by changing the position if movement due to periodontal disease has occurred. Such dentures are provided at the time of extraction and the patient adapts to the new denture.

*Disadvantages* | Requires good cooperation of the patient with the need for close clinical supervision. Alveolar bone resorption occurs rapidly leading to loss of adaptation. After care may require many visits including relines/rebases and replacement dentures. This leads to an increased cost. The clinician is not able to assess trial dentures.

*Procedure* | Initial treatment should be aimed at conservation of the teeth and periodontal treatment. Impressions are taken and the jaw registration is recorded. If edentulous spaces exist then a trial stage is feasible. Casts are prepared to accept those teeth to be extracted. Finally teeth are extracted (Fig. 78) and the dentures placed immediately over the sockets (Fig. 79).

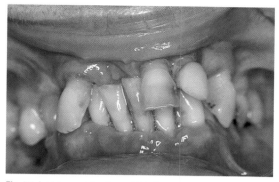

**Fig. 77** A case requiring immediate dentures.

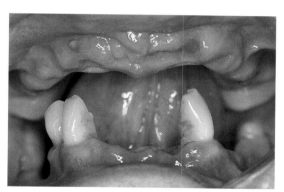

**Fig. 78** Completion of the extractions.

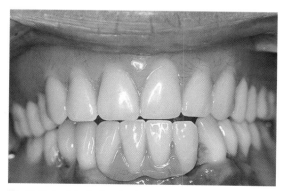

**Fig. 79** Immediate denture in place.

## The denture space impression

*Definition*

The neutral zone is that in which the forces of the cheeks and lips are said to be equalised by those of the tongue; it is also often described as being the zone of minimal conflict.

*Indications*

- Postextraction changes which may make it impossible to determine accurately the former position of the natural teeth.
- Patients who have not worn a lower denture for many years and whose lower lip has collapsed inwards and whose tongue has expanded into the denture space.
- Patients who have very atrophic ridges such that the stability of the denture is dependent on muscular control.
- Mandibular resections resulting in differing anatomical architecture of the region and modified tongue movements.
- Parkinson's disease or situations where muscle tone and movements have altered.

*Advantages*

A base plate (Figs 80, 81 & 82) is used to record the buccal and lingual polished surfaces during the impression technique. The eventual tooth position is in an area where the buccal and lingual forces tending to displace the denture are in reciprocal equilibrium. The final denture therefore tends to be better tolerated.

*Disadvantages*

The procedure is technique sensitive and requires a cooperative patient.

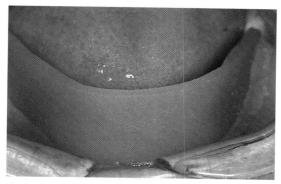

**Fig. 80** Vertical fin tray in mouth.

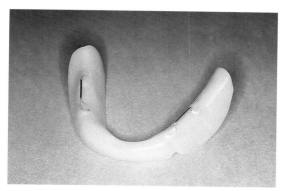

**Fig. 81** Baseplate with retentive spurs.

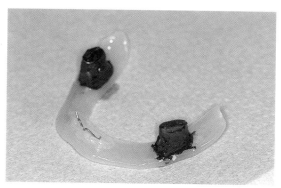

**Fig. 82** Baseplate with greenstick occlusal pillars.

## Resection case

*Definition*

A patient who has had a mandibular resection (Fig. 83) with altered anatomical architecture of the region and possible sensory and motor nerve damage to this area and surrounding structures.

*Indications*

A tethered tongue or abnormal movements of the tongue caused by motor nerve damage which can result in instability of a lower denture.

*Advantages*

Patients who have had radical surgery for oral cancer want to return to 'normality' as soon as possible, both aesthetically and functionally. Many of these patients previously were considered to be poor candidates for prosthetic rehabilitation. However the neutral zone technique allows the placement of a lower denture in a number of these cases; the denture to be constructed has to allow for the changes in architecture and muscle tone that have resulted from this type of surgery (Figs 84 & 85). Patients receiving this treatment may also require the use of implants to help with denture retention.

*Disadvantages*

Skin grafts or postsurgical radiotherapy can complicate the placement of a prosthesis in this region. Skin can react in a different manner to oral mucosa when subjected to denture loading.

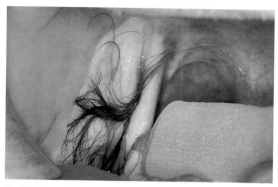

**Fig. 83** Resected mandible with skin graft.

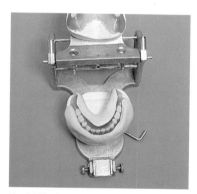

**Fig. 84** Teeth position relative to neutral zone template.

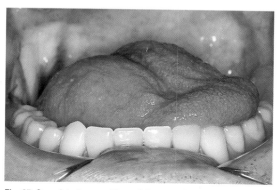

**Fig. 85** Completed case with teeth in neutral zone.

## Clinical application of a neutral zone technique

*Definition*

As given previously.

*Materials*

One of the baseplates as shown (in Figs 80 & 81, p 56). The impression material will be either a tissue conditioner or an addition silicone putty material depending on the base chosen. The use of a viscoelastic material allows for better moulding of the material to take place during function over an extended time. The use of an impression material has the limitation of its shorter setting time and flow characteristics.

*Procedure*

1. The base is placed in the mouth and its stability checked. Any modification to the base or fin are undertaken at this stage.
2. The height of the fin is adjusted to the desired occlusal face height for the patient.
3. The denture space impression material is placed lateral and medial to the fin and the patient is asked to 'pout' in order to mould the buccal periphery and then asked to perform various tongue movements to mould the lingual surface.
4. The technician then pours plaster or silicone jigs of this denture space impression (Fig. 86) and a wax rim is constructed into this region.
5. The teeth are set-up within the constraints of the jigs and the width of teeth modified as required (Figs 87 & 88).

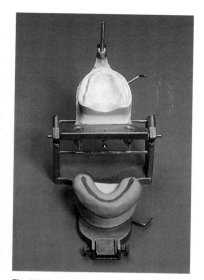

**Fig. 86** Neutral zone template.

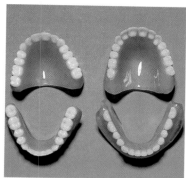

**Fig. 87** Comparison of old and neutral zone dentures.

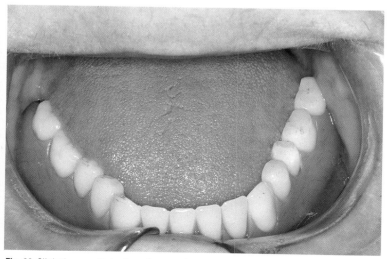

**Fig. 88** Clinical case with teeth set in neutral zone.

## Hollow glove technique

*Definition*

An obturator is a prosthetic appliance that closes or obturates an opening. The opening is commonly a maxillary defect (Fig. 89) that is either congenital in origin, such as a cleft palate, or surgically traumatic such as a hemimaxillectomy.

*Indications*

This technique is indicated where a large defect exists and where the retention of the prosthesis may well be a problem due to its size. This obturator is made in two parts; the elastic obturator portion can be placed into the defect utilising any undercut present to aid with retention of the oral prosthesis. This type of appliance can also be used for smaller defects where the elastic nature of the material will aid in retention of the prosthesis.

*Advantages*

This technique allows for obturation of the majority of the defect because of the elastic nature of the material used—most commonly a resilient lining material. It therefore provides a better seal, preventing nasal secretions into the oral cavity and air leakage from one compartment to the other.

*Disadvantages*

The technique does not provide as much soft tissue support to the cheek as a rigid obturator will. If the malar has been resected the final appearance may be compromised.

*Procedure*

A base plate (Fig. 91) is made in the laboratory and added to this is the elastic obturator (Fig. 90) which clips onto a rim of heat-cured acrylic or utilises magnets to adhere to the prosthesis.

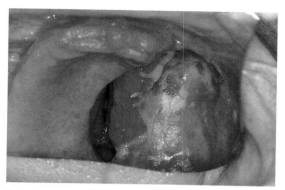

**Fig. 89** Large palatal defect.

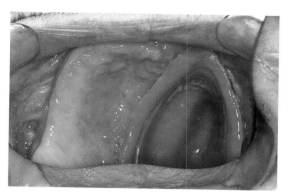

**Fig. 90** First part of obturator (hollow glove).

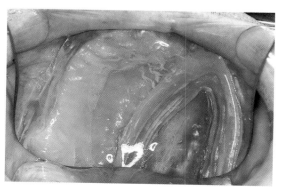

**Fig. 91** Clear baseplate covers palate and links into glove.

## Hollow box obturator

*Definition*

A hollow box or hollow bulb made in heat-cured acrylic; the acrylic filling the maxillary defect is left hollow.

*Indications*

To fill a maxillary defect (Fig. 92) and support the soft tissue walls of the region; this type of denture is preferable to other appliances.

*Advantages*

The use of such a technique reduces the weight of the maxillary prosthesis (Fig. 93) allowing considerably improved retention (Fig. 94).

*Disadvantages*

- If the maxillary defect is large and involves the floor of the orbit, the size of a one-piece obturator, coupled with the trismus that is present in some resection patients, may make placement of such a prosthesis difficult.
- The flasking of such a large appliance can be difficult and the subsequent addition of the palatal polished surface requires an additional laboratory procedure.

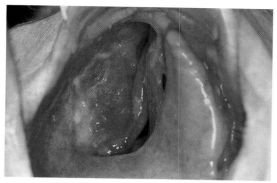

**Fig. 92** Right Hemimaxillectomy.

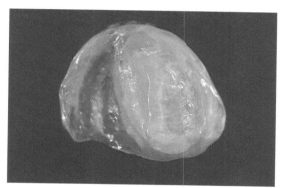

**Fig. 93** One-piece obturator with a hollow bung.

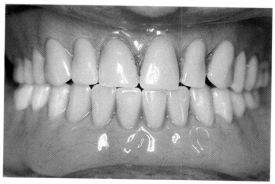

**Fig. 94** Completed denture in place.

## Acrylic surface

*Definition*

An acrylic appliance designed to cover the occlusal and/or incisal surfaces of the teeth to refine and/or correct the occlusion present (Fig. 95).

*Indications*

Where an onlay is required in the anterior region, and an overdenture may be difficult to place due to undercuts, the use of a tooth-coloured resin material can provide both a pleasing and functional result. The use of acrylic resin in the posterior region, which is required as a functional necessity, may also provide enhanced appearance (Figs 96 & 97).

*Advantages*

The use of a tooth-coloured removable appliance in the anterior region of the mouth to replace tooth substance loss is often a simpler approach than the more advanced fixed restorative procedures.

*Disadvantages*

Acrylic is a weak material and may not be of sufficient strength to withstand the occlusal loading. It is prone to breakage and has to be bulky to gain adequate strength.

*Management*

The use of acrylic material to compensate for tooth substance loss has certain advantages. However the cause of the tissue loss should be addressed prior to placement of such an appliance, otherwise subsequent wear of the acrylic will occur.

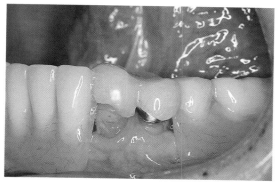

**Fig. 95** Denture onlayed on worn premolar teeth.

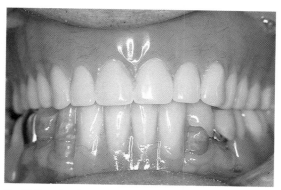

**Fig. 96** Completed case—anterior view.

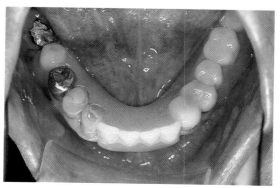

**Fig. 97** Completed case—occlusal surface.

## Acrylic/composite resin

*Definition*

An acrylic or composite resin moulded to cover the incisal or occlusal surfaces of the teeth to refine/correct the occlusion present and improve the appearance (Figs 98, 99 & 100).

*Indications*

Hypodontia and cases of tooth substance loss. The purpose of a removable prosthesis is that the change in occlusal face height can be evaluated with such treatment, and the aesthetic result can be assessed.

*Advantages*

The use of a tooth-coloured material in a removable appliance in the anterior region of the mouth to replace tooth substance loss is often simpler than more advanced fixed restorative procedures. This type of restoration compared to a fixed design offers considerable savings both in finance and time.

*Disadvantage*

The junction of natural tooth to acrylic is difficult to hide.

*Procedure*

Because of the disadvantage (see above) an assessment of the patient's lip line is important. The use of composite resin to construct the onlay gives an improved appearance and also allows a better junction to be constructed. The use of 4-Meta adhesives has meant that mechanical retention to the denture alloy is no longer necessary and therefore the onlay can be made thinner and less unsightly. This simplifies the procedure, as the casting needs only sandblasting prior to bonding agents being applied.

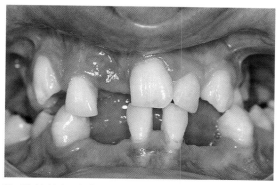

**Fig. 98** Multiple missing units and malalignment.

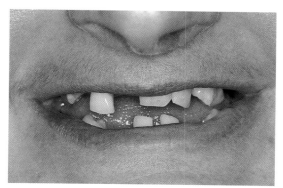

**Fig. 99** Existing appearance.

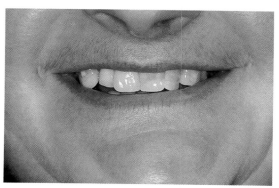

**Fig. 100** Acrylic anterior onlay partial denture.

## Cobalt/chrome surface

*Definition*

An onlay denture is designed to alter the shape and height of the occlusal surfaces of the teeth over which it fits. It may be constructed of: acrylic resin, gold, stainless steel or cobalt chromium alloy.

*Indications*

Where there is a need to improve the occlusal contact of teeth; or where the appliance will increase the occlusal vertical dimension until it is similar to that which was present before tooth substance loss occurred (Figs 101, 102 & 103).

*Advantages*

A cast metal surface is present in the posterior segments which will provide a robust occlusion for functional purposes.

*Disadvantages*

If the patient is a severe bruxist and cobalt chromium onlays are used there is the potential for the opposing dentition to be worn down. The appearance of metal onlay appliances may also preclude their use.

*Procedure*

1. The patient is provided with a temporary acrylic appliance to increase the occlusal vertical dimension to the required height. This is worn for a period of time in order to assess compliance.
2. If the appliance is clinically satisfactory then a face-bow mounting on an arcon articulator is used to mount the master casts, allowing the increase in vertical dimension to be waxed up before casting.
3. The occlusion can be refined intraorally.

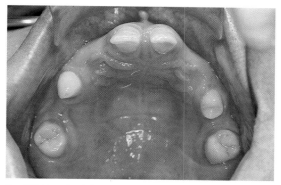

**Fig. 101** Hypodontia in upper arch.

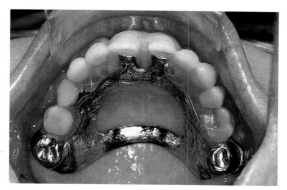

**Fig. 102** Replacement of teeth with CoCr onlay denture.

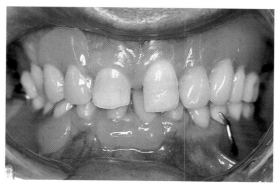

**Fig. 103** Completed case—anterior view.

## Every denture

*Definition*

A mucosa-borne denture that conforms to a specific design to ensure gingival health. It is restricted to the upper arch (Fig. 104).

*Design*

The denture requires the presence of bounded saddles. The design should incorporate the following points:
- Point contact between natural and artificial teeth
- Wide embrasures
- 'Free-occlusion'
- Uncovered gingivae
- Distal stabilisers (Fig. 105).

General principles of partial denture construction should be followed.

*Advantages*

The open design allows a hygienic denture to be constructed which is retentive and stable and minimises damage to the supporting and surrounding tissues.

*Disadvantages*

It does require the presence of bounded saddles so that the point contact can be maintained throughout the archform. Even where the most distal tooth is missing however, 'Every principles' can still be incorporated into the denture design.

*Procedure*

The construction of the denture follows normal prosthetic technique. An accurate impression is required to establish the point contact between the teeth. Originally porcelain teeth were advocated but, due to their expense and low availability, acrylic teeth are now used. The distal stabilisers are not clasps and are constructed from wrought stainless steel to contact the distal surface of the most posterior teeth and maintain interproximal contact (Fig. 106).

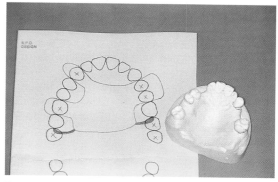

**Fig. 104** Every denture design.

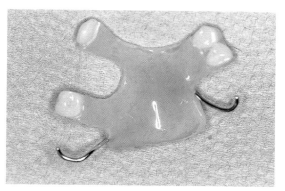

**Fig. 105** Every acrylic denture with distal stabilisers.

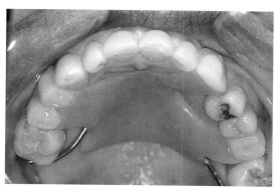

**Fig. 106** Completed Every denture.

# Spoon design upper denture

*Definition*

A simple acrylic denture made to replace one or two anterior teeth (Figs 107, 108 & 109). It derives its support entirely from the anterior ridge and palate.

*Indications*

Where a patient has suffered the loss of one or two anterior teeth. There should be a wide well formed palate with sufficient anterior clearance between the lower incisors and the ridge.

*Advantages*

Spoon dentures are cheap, easy to construct and modify. This has obvious advantages following the initial loss of a single tooth at the front of the mouth.

*Disadvantages*

Such a denture is weak and nonrigid. Therefore it is prone to breakage with continuous wear especially from occlusal forces from the lower anterior teeth. To avoid this, such dentures are sometimes made bulky for strength and this may not be accepted by the patient. Furthermore these dentures are small in size and may be inadvertently swallowed or inhaled. It would prove impossible to track such an object within the body cavities as acrylic is radiolucent. Such dentures therefore should use radiopaque resin to limit medico-legal liability.

*Procedure*

Impressions are taken and the shade and mould selected. Generally the working models can be located without the need for a registration visit. If appearance and occlusion are satisfactory then the denture is processed.

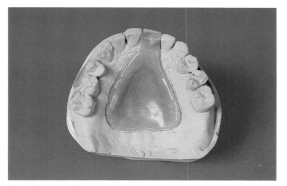

**Fig. 107** Spoon denture during construction.

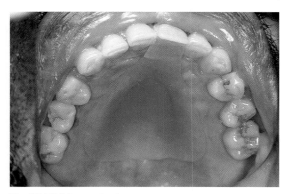

**Fig. 108** Trial denture in place.

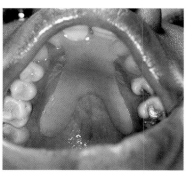

**Fig. 109** Bifid spoon denture in place.

## Acrylic lingual plate versus wrought lingual bar connector

*Definition*

- A partial acrylic lower denture may be constructed as an all acrylic prosthesis.
- The anterior connector may incorporate the use of a wrought metal bar.

*Indications*

The acrylic lingual plate connector is used commonly as it is technically less demanding and provides increased tooth support to the prosthesis (Figs 110 & 111). Where there is sufficient space a wrought lingual bar should take preference, as this design is periodontally more favourable (Fig. 112).

*Advantages*

- The acrylic lingual plate connector has the advantage of being easy to construct and modify. It is also less costly in laboratory time.
- The wrought metal connector is less obtrusive to the patient and does not cover the gingival tissues. It is also stronger and less bulky than the acrylic connector.

*Disadvantages*

- The acrylic connector will cover the gingival margins and may cause damage by:
  — mechanical stripping of the gingivae
  — interdental wedging
  — encouraging plaque formation on the teeth.
- The main disadvantage of the wrought metal connector is the increased technical cost involved in production. Insufficient depth of the lingual sulcus may also prevent the use of the bar.

*Procedure*

*For the acrylic lingual plate connector* it is important to avoid contact with the gingiva and obtain relief by blocking out the dentogingival junction, in addition to any interdental spaces on the cast. The aim is to reduce coverage of gingival margins where possible.

*The wrought bar* is constructed from preformed wrought stainless steel bars that can be cold worked to conform to the archform lingually.

Oral hygiene should be of a high standard in both situations.

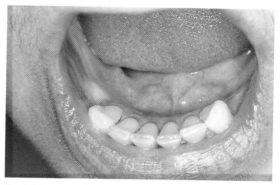

**Fig. 110** Lone standing lower anterior teeth.

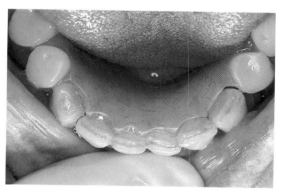

**Fig. 111** Acrylic lingual connector.

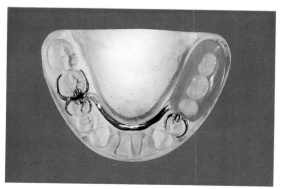

**Fig. 112** Wrought lingual bar connector.

## Wrought clasps to aid with retention

*Definition*

Acrylic partial dentures generally rely on the use of cohesive and adhesive forces of saliva together with the traditional forces associated with full denture retention and stability. To assist this process the clinician may wish to place clasps on the denture (Figs 113, 114 & 115).

*Indications*

Wrought clasps are placed in acrylic dentures to aid retention if potential problems in this area are envisaged.

*Advantages*

Such clasps are relatively easy to place. They can be adjusted at the chairside to help increase the retention.

*Disadvantages*

If not correctly placed relative to the survey line, they may cause gingival damage and will also increase plaque accumulation. If the clasp arm is not correctly adapted it may also cause ulceration in the sulcus.

*Procedure*

A wrought clasp is placed in the correct position on the tooth after the trial denture stage has been completed as its positioning will not be stable in wax. The position of the clasp head and its design must be clearly indicated by the clinician.

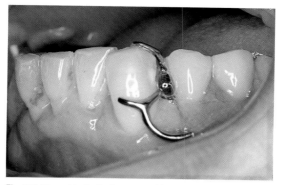

**Fig. 113** Wrought gingivally approaching clasp.

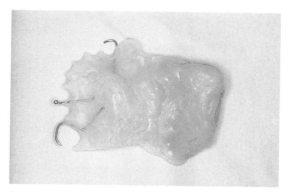

**Fig. 114** Assortment of wrought clasps used to help retain a temporary obturator.

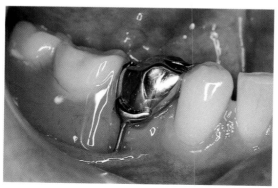

**Fig. 115** Wrought gingivally approaching clasp.

## Conventional type

*Definition*

A cobalt/chromium partial denture allows the prosthesis to incorporate both strength and rigidity. Such a denture may utilise these properties to obtain its support and retention from the natural teeth. When cast in thin sections it may be of sufficient flexibility to make use of undercuts. In thick sections its rigidity will resist deformation (Figs 116, 117 & 118).

*Indications*

Such a denture is indicated where there is good oral hygiene and high patient motivation to accept a prosthesis. Where there is a wide distribution of abutment teeth which have adequate bone support and the clinician wishes to derive the support from the teeth then this type of denture is the one of choice.

*Advantages*

- The extra strength and rigidity, especially in small sections, allow for the manufacture of smaller, less bulky dentures.
- They also have the flexibility when cast in thin sections to allow cast clasps to engage undercuts and obtain retention from the teeth.

*Disadvantages*

- Metal is unsightly and therefore cannot be used at the front of the mouth.
- Cobalt/chromium requires casting and is therefore more costly in terms of laboratory time.

*Procedure*

1. Preliminary casts are mounted and surveyed prior to a decision being made regarding the type of denture that will be provided.
2. The master impression is taken in an elastomeric material and the resultant cast poured in reinforced dental stone.
3. This master cast is then duplicated in investment material and the design is constructed in wax following the clinician's prescription.
4. The casting is made, polished and delivered to the clinician.

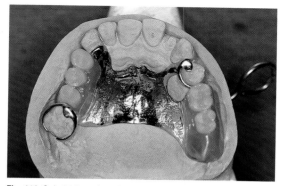

**Fig. 116** Cobalt/chromium denture with palatal connector.

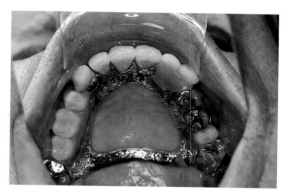

**Fig. 117** Cobalt/chromium denture with anterior and palatal bar connector.

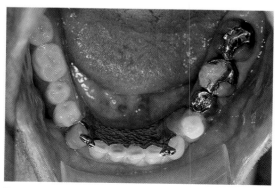

**Fig. 118** Cobalt/chromium denture with lingual plate.

## Kennedy class IV

*Definition*

A bounded saddle which lies entirely anterior to the abutment teeth (Figs 119, 120 & 121). It has no modifications but the length of saddle may vary from a single tooth to multiple units.

*Indications*

The treatment indicated depends on the individual patient, and can involve the provision of a bridge or an implant. The criteria for which treatment modality is indicated depends on such factors as: if the abutment teeth are of poor coronal form or not amenable to crowning for bridgework, or gross alveolar resorption making implant placement difficult. The use of a cobalt/chromium denture would therefore be indicated to replace missing anterior units.

*Advantages*

- A cobalt/chromium denture offers strength, especially where there is limited space between the opposing teeth and the ridge.
- The use of cobalt/chromium backings can also help in cases of bruxism in order to prevent fracture of the anterior saddle arèa.
- Support for the denture can be gained from the abutment teeth on either side of the saddle.
- The design may also involve the posterior teeth for further support.

*Disadvantages*

- The forward position of the saddle makes indirect retention of the denture a problem. The design uses support from the posterior teeth and retentive clasps are placed on the molar teeth. The clasp axis will be posteriorly placed and allow rotation of the anterior saddle during function. To prevent this, indirect retainers are placed on the most posterior teeth or the palatal connector is extended towards the soft palate. If this is not possible then the lack of indirect retention will be a problem.
- Unlike acrylic dentures, cobalt/chromium does not produce a good adhesive seal between itself, saliva and the oral mucosa.

*Procedure*

1. The cast is surveyed with an appropriate design which must consider the problems of support together with direct and indirect retention.
2. A path of insertion may also be considered to utilise the anterior buccal undercut present.

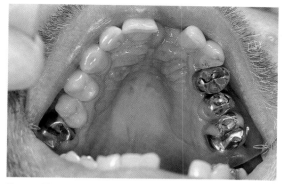

**Fig. 119** Missing anterior incisor.

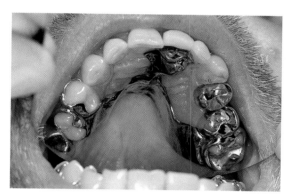

**Fig. 120** Replacement with cobalt/chromium denture.

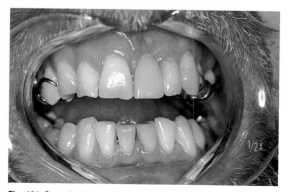

**Fig. 121** Completed case.

## Lower swinglock

A cobalt/chromium plate which has a hinge and lock which allows the utilisation of naturally occurring hard and soft tissue undercuts in the retention of a partial denture (Fig. 122).

- Inadequate support; teeth which could not normally support a partial denture can be utilised in a swinglock design.
- Missing key abutments; the transmission of forces to the remaining dentition is fundamental.
- Inadequate retention; the use of previously unavailable undercuts by this design allows for increased retention.
- Maxillofacial prosthesis; the retention and stability of such a prosthesis is enhanced by the swinglock design.

- Shallow vestibule.
- Extended fraenum.
- Aesthetic considerations.
- Occlusal interferences.
- Poor plaque control.

1. A master impression is taken making sure that the full functional depth of the sulcus is recorded in the dentate region where the swinglock arm is going to gain retention.
2. A decision is made as to which side the hinge and lock (Fig. 123) will be positioned.
3. The cobalt/chromium casting is produced and tried in (Fig. 124).

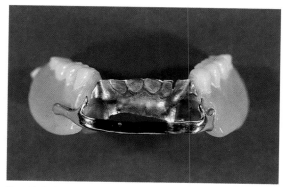

**Fig. 122** Swinglock denture showing anterior bar.

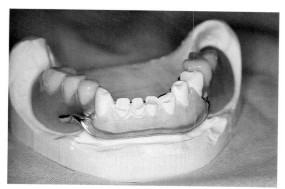

**Fig. 123** Locked in position on cast.

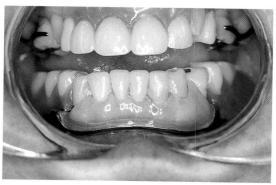

**Fig. 124** Completed case.

# Rotational path of insertion

*Definition*

Krol describes a rotational path prosthesis which seats its first segment, containing the centres of rotation, followed by the remaining framework which is rotated into position thus locating the second segment to the final position of the prosthesis. Two classifications are described:
- Category 1 includes all prostheses that have postero-anterior paths of insertion or anteroposterior paths replacing posterior segments.
- Category 2 includes all lateral paths and anteroposterior paths replacing anterior segments.

*Indications*

This technique can be utilised particularly in Kennedy Class IV situations where the clasping of anterior abutment teeth can be unsightly. The technique also offers an alternative to the principle of guide surfaces where minimal naturally occurring undercuts may exist.

*Advantages*

Tooth coverage is reduced making plaque control easier, affecting both the caries rate and periodontal health. Appearance can be improved without the need to resort to precision attachments or clasping of anterior teeth.

*Disadvantages*

The complexity of the design and the surveying principles involved in paralleling the rest seat walls to the proximal retentive surface make this technique both clinically and technically demanding.

*Procedure*

The analysis of undercuts is carried out as normal using a traditional surveyor (Fig. 125); further analysis is done using a divider to assess the path of rotation.
In this category 2 situation, the rigid proximal retainer is seated first and the posterior retainers are rotated into position (Figs 126 & 127).

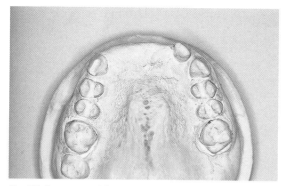

**Fig. 125** Cast surveyed for rotation insertion.

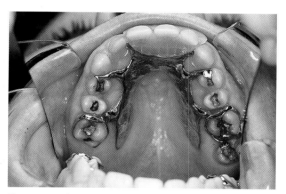

**Fig. 126** Upper occlusal view of partial denture.

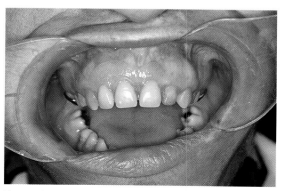

**Fig. 127** Anterior view of partial denture.

# Altered cast technique

Technique to obtain a selective impression of the differential support offered by the free end saddle. The objective is to obtain a displacive impression of the edentulous under conditions which mimic functional loading.

*Indications*

A cobalt/chromium partial denture constructed for a free end saddle will need the differential support offered by the abutment tooth which is relatively rigid in its socket, supported by the periodontal ligament and the more displaceable denture bearing mucosa. The use of the altered cast technique therefore takes into account the differential support provided by oral mucosa and teeth.

*Advantages*

- Better support for the free end saddle as the impression of the tissues is taken under conditions which mimic functional load.
- It may also help to redefine the extensions of the saddle following the master impression.

*Disadvantages*

- The original technique described by Applegate used special functional impression waxes which allowed moulding of the tissues under load.
- The technique may also disrupt the occlusal positioning of the teeth if it is undertaken as a rebasing of the finished denture, leading to considerable adjustment at the chairside.

*Procedure*

1. A cobalt/chromium framework is designed in a conventional fashion (Fig. 128) and an acrylic close fitting tray is added to it (Fig. 129).
2. An impression is taken using either zinc oxide/eugenol paste or a medium viscosity silicone impression material.
3. When the framework is placed in the mouth the impression is taken with finger pressure applied to the occlusal rests of the cobalt/chromium framework.
4. The set impression is removed from the mouth and reseated on the master cast which has had the edentulous areas removed.
5. The new impression is poured and a composite cast is produced (Fig. 130).

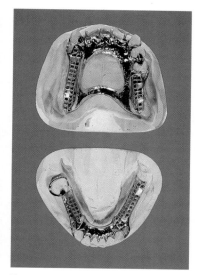

**Fig. 128** Cobalt/chromium framework for free end saddle.

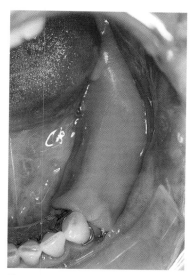

**Fig. 129** Close fitting special tray in position.

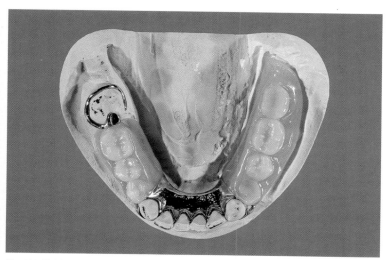

**Fig. 130** Finished denture on altered cast.

## Lingual swinglock

*Definition*

A cobalt/chromium casting with a hinge and lock arrangement to utilise the naturally occurring lingual undercuts in the lingual sulcus of a partially dentate individual for the retention of a prosthesis.

*Indications*

In the posterior mandible, deep lingual undercuts (Fig. 131) often present a design problem in a partial denture situation where the use of these areas is somewhat restricted by the bilateral application. Changing the path of insertion may allow utilisation of one of these areas. However a two-part design or swinglock principle is needed to make use of both regions (Fig. 132).

*Advantages*

This allows full extension of the denture into the functional lingual sulcus and thereby gives both increased support and retention to the prosthesis as well as maximising the lateral bracing provided (Fig. 133).

*Disadvantages*

- The placement of such a prosthesis can be a problem depending on where the hinge and lock come in the arch form. The degree to which the gate can open is somewhat limited as the tongue can interfere with this opening.
- Poor plaque control is also commonly found in this region and therefore may be exacerbated by the placement of such a design.

*Procedure*

An accurate impression is taken using an elastic impression material but often the extent of the undercuts necessitates a two-part impression technique.

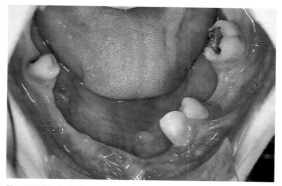

**Fig. 131** Clinical view showing severity of lingual undercut.

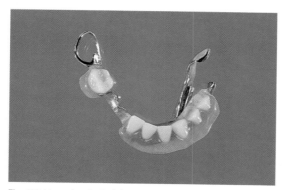

**Fig. 132** Lingual swinglock in open position.

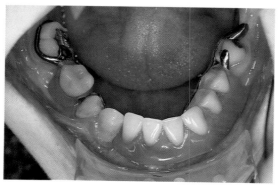

**Fig. 133** Swinglock denture in place.

## Split pin

*Definitions*

- A sectional denture is constructed in two parts that link together and utilise the undercut areas to aid retention.
- A split pin and hollow tubing may be used to retain the two parts of a sectional denture together.

*Indications*

Sectional dentures are able to utilise undercuts around the teeth and associated soft and hard tissues which would not be available to a conventional partial denture which used one path of insertion and removal. A split pin occupies less space than the incorporation of a lock and bolt and this therefore looks better especially in the replacement of anterior saddles (Fig. 134).

*Advantages*

The split pin arrangement is small and therefore can be used at the front of the mouth. It is technically easier to construct than the lock and bolt.

*Disadvantages*

The continual frictional contact between the pins and the hollow cylinder results in wear and eventually the retention is lost. This may be remedied by forcing the pins apart to reactivate them.

*Procedure*

1. An accurate recording of the hard and soft tissues, correctly duplicating the undercuts present is required.
2. The position and angulation of the split pins in relation to the occlusion and path of insertion of the second unit needs to be prepared using a parallelometer.
3. The split pin which is cast as part of the cobalt/chrome framework makes frictional contact within a hollow metal tube which is contained within the acrylic portion of the denture (Figs 135 & 136).

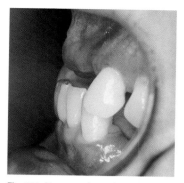

**Fig. 134** Close-up of anterior bounded saddle.

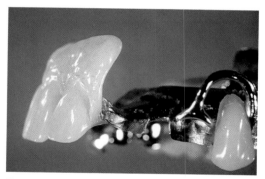

**Fig. 135** Acrylic section attached.

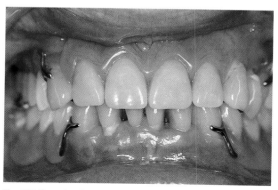

**Fig. 136** Completed case—anterior view.

# Locking bolts

A lock and bolt design is another means of holding together a sectional denture which is constructed in different parts, each with its own path of insertion and removal.

A bounded edentulous span where bridgework is unsuitable either because of the length of the span or the unsuitability of the abutment teeth. The study casts may be rotated or tilted and this would result in potentially useful undercut regions that could be utilised by such a design of denture.

This type of sectional denture is extremely retentive as the two linked portions cannot be removed unless the locking mechanism is released. The locking design means that less occlusal clearance is required than for a split pin sectional denture.

These are related to the increased bulk of the system and the space required to accommodate it. It is generally more demanding technically and this leads to increased cost.

The locking bolt can either be purchased as a complete unit or it can be fabricated in the laboratory. The locking of the bolt can be extremely precise and often a small clip is required to assist the patient with the unlocking of the mechanism (Figs 137, 138 & 139).

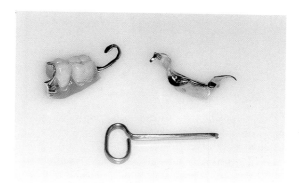

**Fig. 137** Exploded view with key.

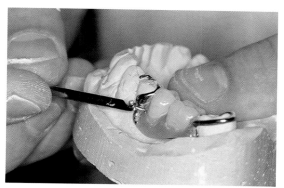

**Fig. 138** Use of key to unlock bolt.

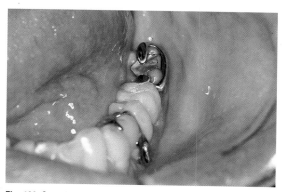

**Fig. 139** Completed case.

## Magnets

*Indication*

Some metal alloys possess magnetic properties which can be utilised in the retention of overdentures or partial dentures (Fig. 140).

*Materials*

Two different alloys are used as magnets in dentistry. These are cobalt-samarium and iron-neodymium-boron. Both of these rare earth magnets have strong attractive forces.

*Advantages*

There is less need for parallel abutments as a rigid line of insertion is not critical. Furthermore, the technique is simple, involving minimal time at the chairside and in the laboratory.

*Disadvantages*

Magnets are brittle materials with a low corrosion resistance. Even when encapsulated in stainless steel, titanium or palladium, the coating may wear and the magnetic alloy will come into contact with saliva. The combination of saliva contact and wear has a deleterious effect on the corrosion resistance of the material.

*Procedure*

- The magnets are placed on the replica of the keepers (Fig. 141) and cured within the denture base material. The overdenture abutments have a cast magnetic alloy post and coping which is placed in the root canal. A direct pick up technique can be used at the chairside where the magnets are directly attached to the denture with autopolymerising acrylic (Fig. 142).
- The stainless steel capsule containing the magnets must be checked regularly as, if this is breached, the magnet will corrode and lose its magnetic properties.

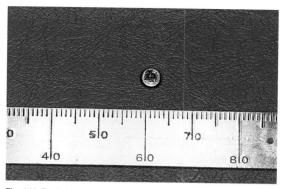

**Fig. 140** Dental magnet.

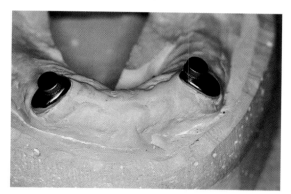

**Fig. 141** Magnets on stone replicas of the keepers.

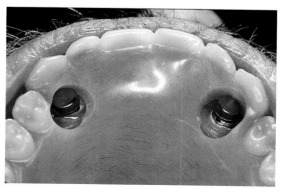

**Fig. 142** Clinical technique for attaching magnets.

## Stud attachment

*Definition*

A ball and socket type of stud attachment in two halves (Fig. 143); the patrix is a circular piece onto which clips the matrix (Fig. 144). The matrix can be reactivated or replaced if it wears with use.

*Advantages*

This mechanism allows an overdenture to be retained on the abutment root face. It provides increased retention to the overdenture. The matrix can either be reactivated if it is a split metal-based cap, or replaced if it is made of a synthetic product.

*Disadvantages*

- When the overdenture is not in place (e.g. overnight) the patrix projects from the root face and can irritate or damage the tongue.
- An adequate space is required within the denture base to house the size of this attachment.
- The leverage applied by such an attachment to the abutment tooth is increased.

*Procedure*

The patrix can be either cast or soldered onto a cast post, although prefabricated posts and patrices are now available. These are cemented within the previously prepared root canal and the matrix is cured within the denture base (Fig. 145). This can either be done in the laboratory or at the chairside, depending on the preference of the clinician.

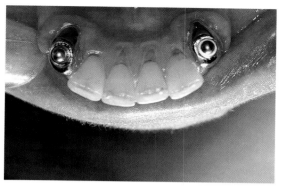

**Fig. 143** Dalbo studs—occlusal view.

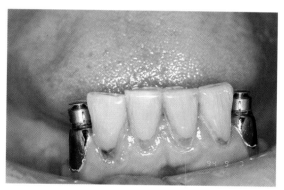

**Fig. 144** Dalbo studs—anterior view with patrix seated.

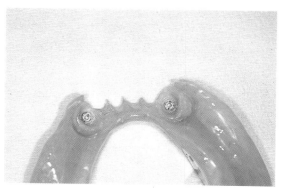

**Fig. 145** Denture with patrix in place.

## Zest anchor attachment

*Definition*

A modification of the ball and socket attachment but, unlike many similar attachments, the socket is seated within the root face (Fig. 146) and the stud attached to the denture base.

*Indications*

- A transitonal aid to provide increased retention while a patient is adapting to a new prosthesis.
- A permanent attachment system if the correct case selection is made.

*Advantages*

- No projection is present from the abutment tooth when the prosthesis is removed.
- The placement of the matrix within the root face is simple and avoids major problems such as two or more retainers needing to be parallel to each other.
- The simple chairside kit is relatively inexpensive and thus of major benefit to the clinician.
- Replacement of the component parts is easy and affordable.

*Disadvantages*

- The use of such an attachment in a bruxist is contraindicated. Patrices wear, particularly if the angulation of the abutments is significantly greater than 15 degrees.
- There is a risk of caries or periodontal breakdown if the patient is not carefully monitored.

*Procedure*

1. The root face is prepared using the latch-grip bur provided in the kit and the prefabricated metal retainer is cemented into the root face using a glass ionomer luting cement.
2. The patrix is then placed within the matrix (Fig. 147) and incorporated directly within the denture using an autopolymerising acrylic resin (Fig. 148).

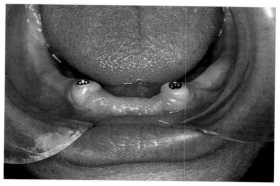

**Fig. 146** Patrix present on root face.

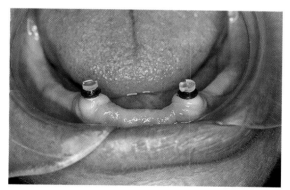

**Fig. 147** Zest attachments on teeth.

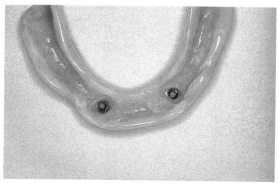

**Fig. 148** Male part in denture.

## Bar attachment

*Definition*

A bar which can be connected between two or more abutment teeth or implants. The shape of the bar can be varied and can be either round, parallel-sided or milled and cast to a customised shape (Fig. 149).

*Indications*

If there is a large span between abutment teeth and tooth support is required, then a bar can be used to connect the abutments. A denture can be provided which contains a clip (Fig. 150) allowing accurate location of the overdenture and increased retention and support (Fig. 151).

*Advantages*

The bar provides support and retention for the denture over its entire length. Various shapes of bar are available which provide additional benefits to suit the indications for use, such as lateral stability provided by a parallel-sided bar.

*Disadvantages*

The bar or the clip may wear if made of dissimilar materials. The bar may need to be adapted if the abutment teeth are in a particular position in the arch, e.g. to keep the bar overlying the residual ridge.

*Procedure*

The bar is normally cast using the lost wax technique from prefabricated bar sections which are prepared in the laboratory on the abutment teeth. The clip can be processed in the laboratory or at the chairside.

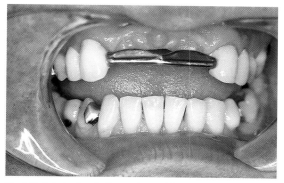

Fig. 149 Anterior bar linking canine and first premolar teeth.

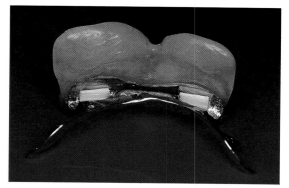

Fig. 150 Hader clips in denture.

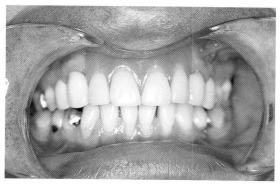

Fig. 151 Denture in place.

# Extracoronal attachment

*Definition*
An attachment involving two parts: the first half has a ball joint or a similar component cantilevered from the abutment unit; the second part, the socket, is housed within the denture base (Fig. 152). This may contain a spring for resilience.

*Indications*
This type of attachment is used in a free-end saddle situation where stress-breaking is a risk (Fig. 153). The patrix is connected to the distal abutment to align with the saddle and allow flexion of this portion in relation to the residual dentition.

*Advantages*
The attachment compensates for the differential compressibility of the supporting structures of the denture base, i.e. the mucosa and teeth. The support provided by abutment teeth and oral mucosa is not equal and would result in instability of the denture base during function.

*Disadvantages*
- This type of attachment requires at least one centimetre of distal crown height of the abutment tooth to be able to house the component parts.
- The extracoronal nature of this attachment results in an altered contour of the abutment tooth which may be difficult to clean (Fig. 154).
- Loss or fracture of the spring housed within the matrix could result in the denture sinking and causing possible damage to the supporting structures.

*Procedure*
This type of attachment involves advanced laboratory support and requires careful clinical assessment of the supporting structures and the occlusion.

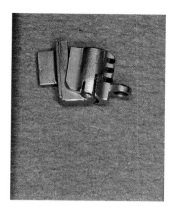

**Fig. 152** Extracoronal attachment.

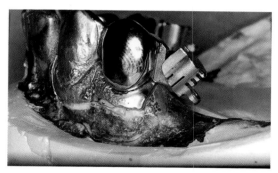

**Fig. 153** Casting incorporating attachment.

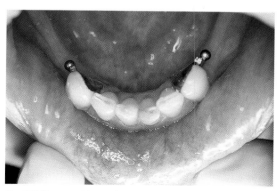

**Fig. 154** Crowns with attachment.

## Ceka attachment

*Definition*

An attachment which has a patrix conical portion with a split head for activation and a matrix cap portion (Figs 155 & 156).

*Indications*

The Ceka attachment was developed as an extracoronal attachment. However, it can also be used for both root face abutments and bars. In the latter case it allows increased retention of the superstructure where a clip may not be provided. If the bar is short the placement of a clip may not be possible and therefore the use of such an adjustable attachment can provide the solution.

*Advantages*

The attachment can be used for many different clinical situations (Fig. 157). The matrix ring retainer can be placed in a variety of locations and the patrix component comes in different forms allowing it to be cast, soldered or bonded into place. The patrix has a cross split allowing for activation of this attachment with wear.

*Disadvantages*

The attachment requires adequate space and the correct angulation relative to the path of insertion of the denture.

*Procedure*

The technical stage of positioning this attachment parallel to the path of insertion of the denture requires the use of a parallelometer.

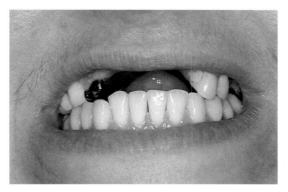

**Fig. 155** Ceka attachment in place.

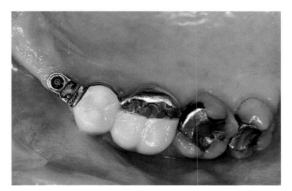

**Fig. 156** Occlusal view.

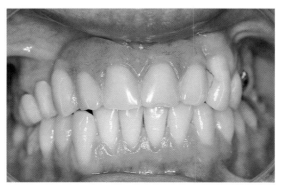

**Fig. 157** Denture in place.

# Intracoronal attachment

*Definition*

As the name suggests, a matrix component part housed within the coronal tissue of the abutment tooth.

*Indications*

- As a resilient intracoronal attachment in the placement of a removable bounded saddle prosthesis (Fig. 159).
- As a nonresilient intracoronal attachment in the fixed movable design of a fixed prosthesis (Fig. 160).

*Advantages*

- The contour of the abutment tooth is not altered as in the extracoronal types.
- In fixed prosthodontics this attachment can overcome the problem of nonparallel abutments.

*Disadvantages*

- The size of this attachment may result in it encroaching upon the pulp chamber, if the tooth is small or pulpal resorption has not occurred.
- Wear of the component parts of a removable prosthesis is inevitable and therefore reactivation is required.
- Adequate preparation of the tooth is required where the component part is to be housed.

*Procedure*

The crown is prepared with the matrix component enclosed within its cast structure. This has to be paralleled to the other portion of the second abutment tooth.

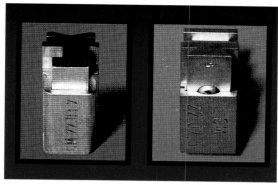

**Fig. 158** Intracoronal attachments.

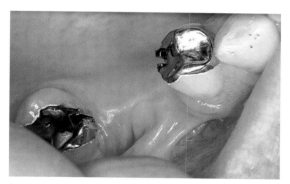

**Fig. 159** Inlays incorporating intracoronal attachments.

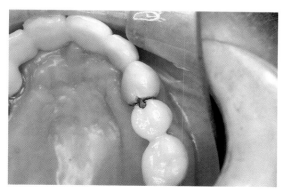

**Fig. 160** A bridge split into smaller units using an intracoronal attachment.

## Abrasion

*Definition*

Loss by wear of tooth substance or a restoration, caused by factors other than tooth contact (Figs 161, 162 & 163).

*Aetiology*

The commonest aetiological agent involved in abrasion is described as resulting from over-vigorous toothbrushing or abrasive dentifrices on exposed dentine. However this is now not thought to be the only mechanism affecting cervical abrasion cavities and chemical erosion may well be an additional factor. Abrasion has been subdivided into:

- two-bodied abrasion, where two surfaces move against each other, e.g. biting or chewing a hair grip or pipestem, and
- three-bodied abrasion where an intervening slurry is at work, e.g. toothpaste or food.

*Management*

The management of tooth surface loss is firstly preventive to stop further deterioration and secondly restorative if the degree of loss necessitates the replacement of the lost tooth substance. Aetiological factors should always be identified and addressed prior to any restorative treatment being instigated.

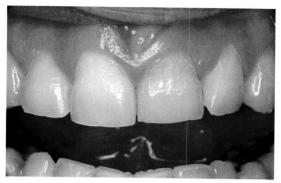

**Fig. 161** Abrasion of upper central incisor.

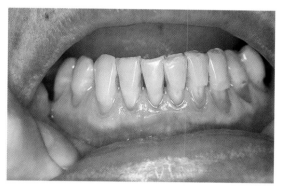

**Fig. 162** Abrasion affecting the cervical margins of all lower left teeth.

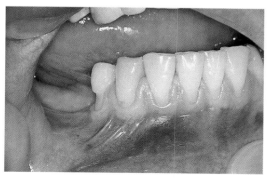

**Fig. 163** Abrasion cavity in the lower right first premolar.

# Attrition

*Definition*

Loss of tooth substance or of a restoration as a result of occlusal or approximal contact between opposing or adjacent teeth (Figs 164 & 165).

*Aetiology*

This type of wear results in the loss of tooth tissue at contacting surfaces. Over a period of time slight wear might be expected at approximal contact points resulting in a flatter, broader contact area. Attrition is often more clearly seen, however, at the occlusal or incisal surfaces of teeth, and such typical wear patterns can be seen clearly in bruxists (Fig. 166). The causes of bruxism are unclear but factors such as stress, uneven occlusal contacts and an habitual tendency have all been suggested.

*Management*

The management of tooth surface loss is firstly preventive to stop further deterioration and secondly restorative if the degree of loss necessitates the replacement of the lost tooth substance.
- The aetiological factors should be identified and addressed prior to any restorative treatment being instigated.
- The use of occlusal appliances to reduce both the damage caused by attrition, and also to restore the lost occlusal vertical dimension in the short term, is the first-line approach in the treatment of this problem.

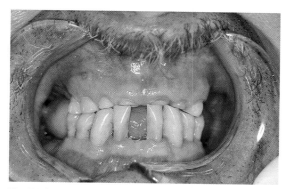

**Fig. 164** Attrition of upper teeth.

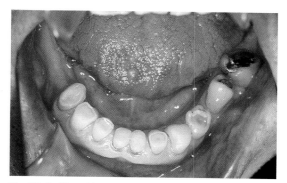

**Fig. 165** Attrition of lower teeth with some erosive element.

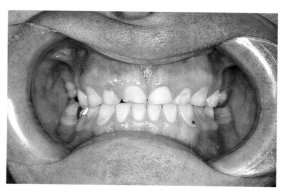

**Fig. 166** Upper and lower arch attrition causing loss of occlusal face height.

## Erosion

*Definition*

Progressive loss of hard dental tissues by a chemical process without bacterial or mechanical action (Fig. 167).

*Aetiology*

Regurgitation and dietary erosion are recognised aetiological factors (Figs 168 & 169). The acidic nature of many foodstuffs or drinks can cause erosion of the dental hard tissues. If a patient suffers from gatrointestinal problems then gastric reflux may result and will produce an acidic oral environment. The clinician should always be aware of erosion caused by anorexia nervosa and bulimia. Other features which influence the erosive effect are the buffering capacity of saliva and medical conditions such as alcoholism.

*Management*

- The aetiological factors implicated in the disease process should be identified and addressed as soon as possible. This preventive approach will stop further deterioration and may obviate the need to restore the eroded tooth surface.
- The restoration of a dentition ravaged by the joint erosive/attrition action is a more commonly encountered problem that demands high levels of restorative skill to resolve.

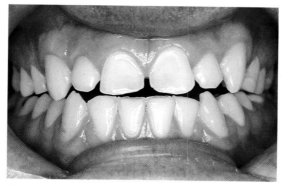

**Fig. 167** Erosion of anterior teeth.

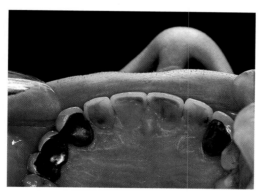

**Fig. 168** Erosion of palatal surfaces of teeth.

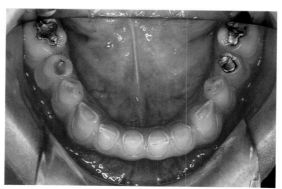

**Fig. 169** Erosion of teeth caused by bulimia.

## Fixed/fixed bridge

*Definition*

A prosthesis where the artificial tooth or teeth (pontic) is supported rigidly on either side by one or more abutment teeth (Figs 170 & 171).

*Indications*

Where missing units are bound by abutment teeth which are capable of supporting the functional load of the missing teeth.

*Advantages*

A fixed/fixed bridge is a strong and retentive restoration for replacing missing teeth. It can be used for single or multiple missing units with the abutment teeth splinted together in the latter case. This can be seen as an advantage as well as a possible disadvantage of this technique as the design of linked abutment units must be considered carefully to allow access for oral hygiene measures.

*Disadvantages*

- This technique requires the preparation of the abutment teeth to be parallel to each other— which may mean: overpreparation of the teeth, structural weakening of the tooth and endangering the pulpal tissues.
- Teeth do move independently in function and this can lead to cementation failure of a fixed/fixed bridge.

*Procedure*

The abutment teeth are prepared with parallel taper (Fig. 172). This can be particularly arduous if the teeth are widely separated, and often means overtapered preparations which are less retentive.

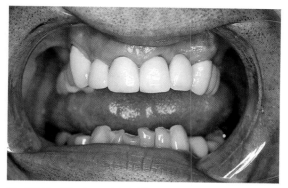

**Fig. 170** Fixed/fixed porcelain bridge.

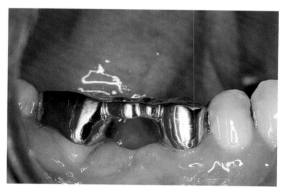

**Fig. 171** Fixed/fixed gold bridge with sanitary pontic design.

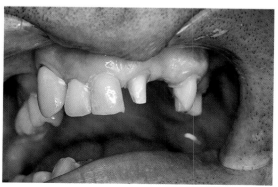

**Fig. 172** Tooth preparation for crown or bridgework.

# Fixed/movable bridge

*Definition*

A prosthesis where the artificial tooth or teeth is rigidly supported on one side, usually the distal end by one or more abutment teeth (Figs 173 & 174). One abutment will contain an intracoronal attachment which allows a small degree of movement between the rigid component and the other abutment tooth or teeth (Fig. 175).

*Indications*

Where abutment teeth are tilted or rotated in relation to each other and the preparation needed to make them parallel would be highly destructive to tooth structure. The construction of large units of bridgework means that the complex task of parallel preparations is increased. The use of movable joints allows for the separation of large units into several smaller more manageable sections.

*Advantages*

Divergent abutments can be used in this technique and are more conservative of tooth structure. Such a bridge allows minor movements of abutments in relation to each other. The parts can be cemented separately.

*Disadvantages*

- This bridge is more demanding of laboratory time leading to increased expense.
- The construction of a temporary bridge is more difficult due to the tilting of the abutment teeth.

*Procedure*

Each abutment tooth can be prepared independently although special consideration should be given to the placement of the movable joint as this is preferably placed intracoronally.

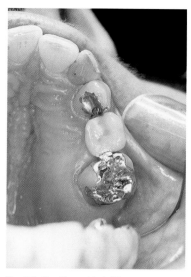

**Fig. 173** Fixed/movable bridge.

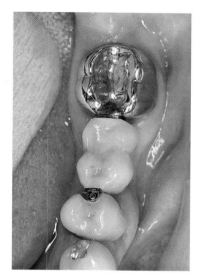

**Fig. 174** Fixed/movable bridge.

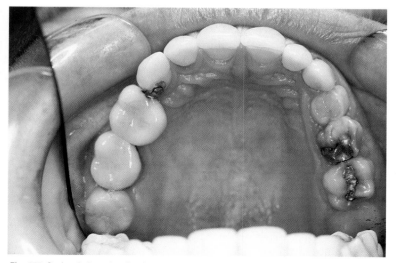

**Fig. 175** Occlusal view showing intracoronal attachment for fixed/movable design.

# Cantilever bridge

*Definition*

A prosthesis where the artificial tooth or teeth are supported on one side only by one or more abutment teeth (Figs 176, 177 & 178).

*Indications*

Where the abutment tooth can carry the occlusal load of the artificial tooth and where the occlusion is protected against potentially demaging rotational forces.

*Advantages*

- This bridge design is generally the most conservative design in terms of tooth preparation (excluding resin retained designs).
- There is no problem of paralleling abutment teeth during preparation.

*Disadvantages*

- The size of pontic is limited to one or two units as leverage forces on the neighbouring abutments can be potentially damaging.
- If a contact point from the pontic to the neighbouring tooth is not placed then potentially rotational forces could be destructive to this type of design.

*Procedure*

A single tooth preparation is carried out on to the abutment tooth in a similar manner to a conventional crown preparation.

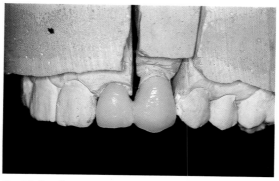

**Fig. 176** Anterior cantilever bridge.

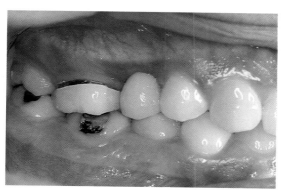

**Fig. 177** Posterior cantilever bridge.

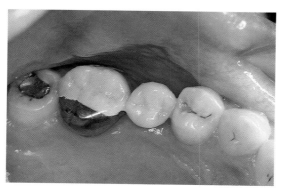

**Fig. 178** Cantilever bridge: occlusal view.

## Spring cantilever bridge

*Definition*

A prosthesis where the artificial tooth is supported by a connecting bar to the abutment tooth or teeth. This connecting arm can be of various lengths depending on the position in the arch of the abutment teeth in relation to the missing unit/s. The arm follows the contour of the palate to allow for patient adaptation (Figs 179, 180 & 181).

*Indications*

This type of restoration is placed where a patient has sound anterior teeth with one missing unit or where diastemas are present around an anterior missing unit.

*Advantages*

- The pontic does not require support from less favourable adjacent teeth.
- Anterior teeth that are sound and might normally be prepared to support a missing unit do not need to be involved. Posterior teeth are more commonly restored than anterior teeth and therefore their use as abutments is less destructive of sound tooth substance.
- Diastemas can be preserved.

*Disadvantages*

- Some patients find the connecting bar in the palate uncomfortable.
- The bar may distort if it is too thin or the occlusion on the pontic is excessive.

*Procedure*

Posterior teeth are prepared for the support of the anterior missing unit. Commonly, the connecting bar does not carry the anterior unit but a core onto which the anterior unit is cemented. This means it can be replaced if the colour needs modification without removing the posterior retainer.

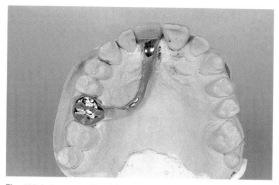

**Fig. 179** Laboratory die with spring cantilever bridge.

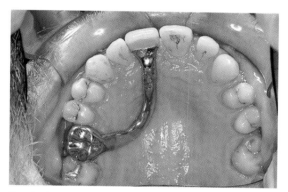

**Fig. 180** Spring cantilever.

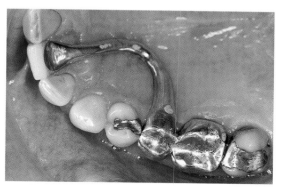

**Fig. 181** Linked abutments for spring cantilever bridge.

# Porcelain jacket and porcelain bonded crown

*Definitions*

- A porcelain jacket crown (PJC) consists of a layer of porcelain which covers the entire crown of the tooth (Fig. 182).
- A porcelain bonded crown (PBC) is one which is constructed in metal alloy with porcelain fused to either all or most of its surfaces (Fig. 182).

*Indications*

- PJC: When the anterior teeth are heavily restored with composite restorations or where tooth material has been lost as a result of trauma.
- PBC: In situations where a stronger restoration is required, such as the presence of minimal interocclusal clearance (Fig. 183).

*Advantages*

- PJC: Improved appearance. The shade and translucency of adjacent teeth can be recreated in porcelain work.
- PBC: The strength of this type of restoration is its major advantage.

*Disadvantages*

- PJC: The brittleness of all-porcelain units and the necessity to remove at least 1 mm of tooth substance are the two main disadvantages of this crown.
- PBC: The necessity to remove at least 1.5 mm of tooth substance buccally to allow for the placement of the alloy and porcelain layers. Unsightliness can result from the difficulty in rendering opaque the alloy layer (Fig. 184).

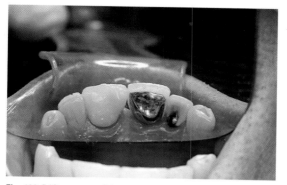

**Fig. 182** PJC on upper right central and PBC on upper left central and lateral.

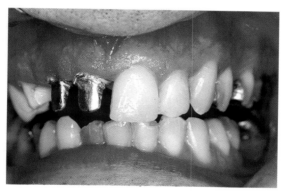

**Fig. 183** Post and core preparations for PBCs.

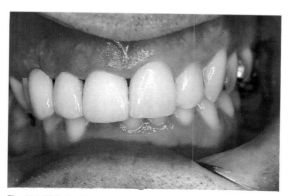

**Fig. 184** PBCs in place.

# Gold veneer crown

*Definition*

A gold veneer or gold shell crown (GSC) is a full veneer crown made of a gold alloy (Figs 185, 186 & 187).

*Indications*

For posterior restorations where appearance is not a consideration. In some cultures a full gold veneer crown on an anterior tooth may denote a sign of wealth or be used as a decorative restoration.

*Advantages*

- Gold can be cast accurately in very thin sections, and can resist repeated loading without distortion.
- Minimal tooth reduction is required when compared to a PBC.
- The incorporation of retention areas for a partial denture, such as rest seats or undercuts, is easily managed with this type of restoration.
- Adhesive gold restorations are now possible by heat treating certain gold alloys to allow adhesive technology to bond the gold to natural tooth structure.

*Disadvantages*

- There are few if any disadvantages of such a restoration other than cost.
- Some people would find it unsightly and its use is therefore mainly limited to posterior units.

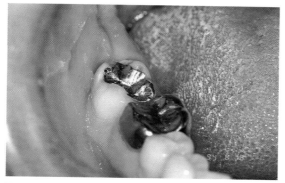

**Fig. 185** Gold crown and simple inlay.

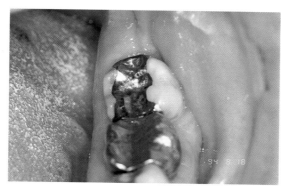

**Fig. 186** Gold crown and complex inlay.

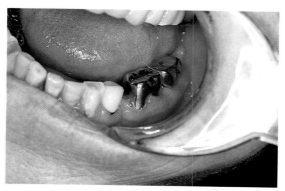

**Fig. 187** Full veneer gold crowns.

# Resin bonded bridge (Maryland)

*Definition*

A prosthesis constructed of a cast metal framework which is luted to the enamel of an abutment tooth by an adhesive composite resin (Figs 188 & 189).

*Indications*

To replace anterior teeth where the abutment teeth are unrestored and the use of conventional bridgework would cause unnecessary tooth destruction.

*Advantages*

Minimal preparation of the abutment tooth is required and is all within enamel, as the retainer is attached to the abutment tooth using acid-etch adhesive techniques.

*Disadvantages*

- These restorations can debond if good isolation is not obtained at the time of cementation.
- If insufficient enamel is present then this type of restoration is unsuitable.
- The restoration is contraindicated where there is evidence of severe tooth wear, parafunction or insufficient interocclusal clearance.

*Procedure*

Cantilevered units are advised (Fig. 190) because if the 'wing retainer' debonds then the bridge will be displaced. Double abutments result in one side debonding but the remaining fixture staying firm. This may lead to caries developing under the debonded retainer. The teeth are prepared with slots or grooves for additional mechanical retention and full lingual coverage to maximise the adhesive bond. The use of a rubber-dam is required to provide the isolation necessary for adhesive bonding techniques.

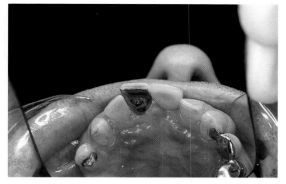

**Fig. 188** Conventional Maryland—upper arch.

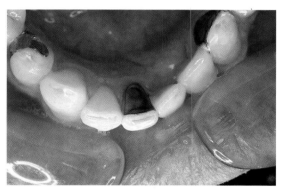

**Fig. 189** Conventional Maryland—lower arch.

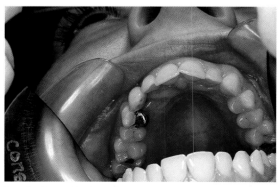

**Fig. 190** Conventional cantilevered Maryland.

# Rochette bridge

*Definition*

An older design of bridge similar to a Maryland bridge, in that it derives its attachment to the abutment tooth using adhesive technology (Figs 191 & 192). The major difference is that the adhesive bond to the metal wing support is mechanical, unlike the chemical and micromechanical adhesion used with a Maryland bridge.

*Indications*

As for a Maryland bridge; however its use is limited and is most often a temporary solution to a failed Maryland bridge.

*Advantages*

- The retention of the composite resin to the metal alloy is mechanical, by counter sunk holes in the retainer. The risk of debonding at the metal/resin interface is dependent on the strength of the resin and not the bond.
- If the restoration does debond recementation is relatively straightforward.

*Disadvantages*

The use of holes in the retainer requires a thicker cross-section of alloy for strength. This may lead to occlusal problems or may feel bulky to the patient.

*Comment*

In the early days of Maryland bridgework debonding was common, initially due to the unpredictable nature of the bond between the alloy and the resin. As a result many of the Maryland bridges were converted to a Rochette design by drilling holes in the retainer (Fig. 192). This often was a poor idea as the metal retainer in a Maryland was much thinner than its predecessor and the retainer was significantly weakened by this technique.

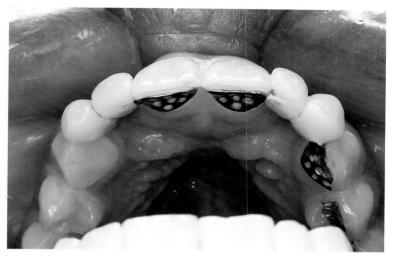

**Fig. 191** Rochette bridge—occlusal view.

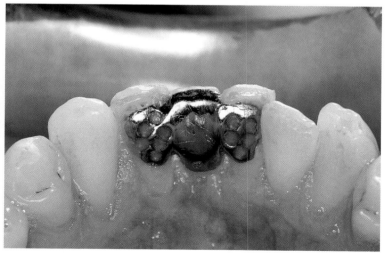

**Fig. 192** Rochette bridge—lingual view.

## Porcelain veneers

*Definition*

A veneer is a thin tooth-shaped porcelain (acrylic or composite) facing cemented to the underlying tooth structure using a filled resin and acid-etch technique to mask discoloured or malformed teeth.

*Indications*

To mask intrinsic staining or surface defects that result in discolouration of anterior teeth (Figs 193 & 194). To correct malformations of tooth shape, spacing (Figs 195 & 196) or tooth chipping due to trauma. Good oral hygiene is essential when considering this type of restoration. A diagnostic wax up to assess the aesthetic result is also advisable.

*Advantages*

Minimal tooth preparation is required. They can provide a superior aesthetic result to full porcelain coverage, as in a PJC, as they allow for some natural tooth colour to show through if desired.

*Disadvantages*

If a substantial amount of natural tooth structure has been lost then a PJC may offer a better alternative as the strength of these restorations is not great. Chipping and cracking of the porcelain because of the thin nature of this restoration can result. This type of restoration is not advised in patients who are bruxists.

*Procedure*

As with all bonding techniques, this procedure is extremely technique sensitive and correct isolation at the time of placement of these restorations is essential.

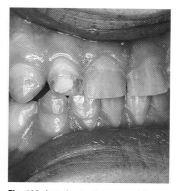

**Fig. 193** Anterior teeth prepared for veneers because of tetracycline staining.

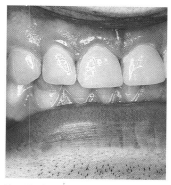

**Fig. 194** Anterior teeth—veneers in place.

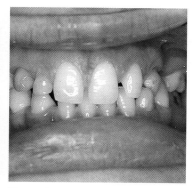

**Fig. 195** Spacing of anterior teeth.

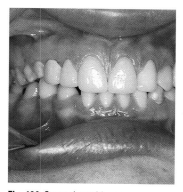

**Fig. 196** Correction with veneers.

# Resin-bonded porcelain crowns

*Definition*

A resin-bonded porcelain crown is a thin section of procelain which encompasses the whole periphery of the tooth unlike a labial or palatal porcelain veneer.

*Indications*

Resin-bonded crowns are indicated for restoring damaged (Fig. 197) or unaesthetic anterior teeth, where a veneer would be inappropriate but a conventional porcelain jacket crown would be too destructive of the remaining tissue.

*Advantages*

These crowns (Figs 198 & 199) require minimal preparation to the tooth. The crown is cemented using adhesive resin technology and, therefore, where diminutive crowns are present there is no advantage to crown lengthening to increase the retention form.

*Disadvantages*

The crown is thin and therefore cannot withstand high occlusal forces. The procedure like so many of the acid-etch techniques is extremely technique sensitive and success is dependent on bonding being carefully followed.

*Procedure*

A reduction of between 0.5 and 0.75 mm should occur allowing adequate enamel to remain for bonding. The incisal region should be reduced by 1 mm to allow enough thickness of porcelain for strength in this region. Margins are preferably produced using a full chamfer and otherwise general crown preparation principles should apply. These include no undercuts or sharp line or point angles.

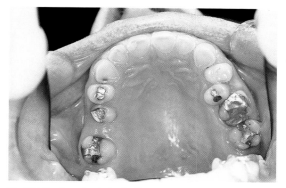

**Fig. 197** Erosion of anterior teeth.

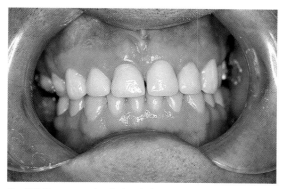

**Fig. 198** Placement of resin-bonded crowns.

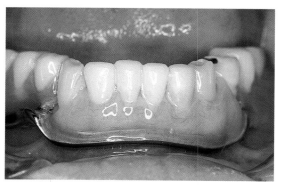

**Fig. 199** Resin-bonded crowns on lower incisors with lower swinglock denture in place.

## Guide surfaces/milled crowns

*Definition*

Two or more parallel surfaces on abutment teeth which limit the path of insertion of a denture. Guide surfaces may occur naturally on teeth or may require to be prepared in the tooth or within a restoration such as an amalgam or gold veneer crown.

*Advantages*

- Increased stability by resisting displacement of the denture.
- Efficient reciprocation of a clasp arm.
- Prevention of clasp deformation during removal of the denture.
- Improvement of the appearance of saddle and tooth (anterior guide surfaces).

*Disadvantages*

The preparation of guide surfaces in the natural dentition will require the removal of tooth substance. However this disadvantage is overcome by the use of naturally occurring guide surfaces or the incorporation of restored teeth.

*Procedure*

- Guide surfaces are produced by removing a minimal and uniform thickness of enamel—usually not more than 0.5 mm—from around the tooth. It should extend vertically for about 3 mm and should be kept as far as possible from the gingival margin.
- The incorporation of a guide surface within a cast restoration may be prepared more accurately with a surveyor in the laboratory (Figs 200, 201 & 202).

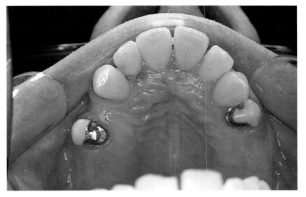

**Fig. 200** Porcelain bonded milled crown.

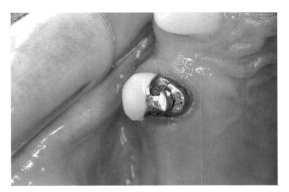

**Fig. 201** Close up of crown.

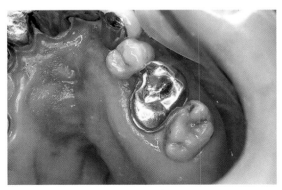

**Fig. 202** Guide surface on gold crown.

## Telescopic crowns

*Definition*

A restoration made in two parts: an inner sleeve of hard gold and an outer full crown which covers this inner unit.

*Indications*

- To overcome differences in the inclination of teeth.
- To provide a removable outer portion for the inspection of the interdental areas or the abutment tooth itself.
- To splint neighbouring teeth.

*Advantages*

The abutment teeth do not require to be parallel and therefore the amount of tooth preparation required is reduced. Removal of the outer crown work is relatively straightforward and allows closer monitoring of the abutment units (Figs 203 & 204).

*Disadvantages*

- Because of the change of the emergence angle of the outer crown from the abutment tooth, particular attention must be paid to plaque removal around the margins.
- The technical stages involved make this more time consuming and therefore more costly than conventional bridgework.

*Procedure*

- The abutment teeth are prepared using conventional procedures and the impression is recorded.
- The inner collars are constructed to allow for a parallel path of insertion for the outer crowns (Figs 205 & 206).

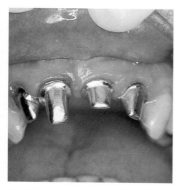

**Fig. 203** Anterior view of telescopic abutments.

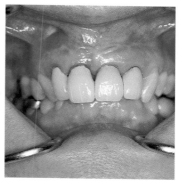

**Fig. 204** Telescopic crowns in place.

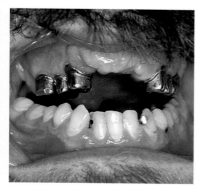

**Fig. 205** Telescopic abutments in place.

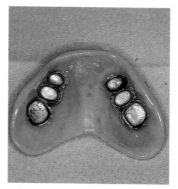

**Fig. 206** Telescopic superstructure incorporated within denture.

## Gold inlays

*Definition*

An intracoronal restoration which is fabricated extraorally and then luted into the prepared cavity.

*Indications*

To give strength in a posterior tooth. Some people prefer gold inlays in anterior teeth, as it is considered aesthetically pleasing or a symbol of wealth.

*Advantages*

- The strength of the alloy when compared to direct restorations.
- The margins of a gold inlay can be thin enough to allow burnishing of the margins intraorally to allow for better marginal adaptation.

*Disadvantages*

The design of an inlay cavity requires that sufficient tooth structure remains to resist the 'wedge' effect. This is where during occlusal loading the inlay creates lateral forces on the walls of the cavity and can result in fractured cusps. Therefore this type of restoration is not suitable for weakened teeth. An onlay design would provide cuspal coverage and prevent the fracture of unsupported tooth tissue (Figs 207 & 208).

*Procedure*

1. The isthmus of the inlay preparation must be no greater than one-third of the intercuspal width or this would result in significant weakening of the tooth.
2. The cavity must not have any undercuts and keep a good retention form.
3. A bevelled margin of approximately 135° is required for gold inlays to allow the feather edge of gold to permit burnishing of the margin (Fig. 209).

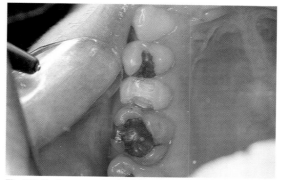

Fig. 207 Tooth preparation for inlay with cuspal coverage.

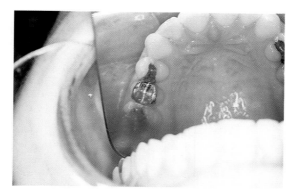

Fig. 208 Cuspal coverage gold inlay.

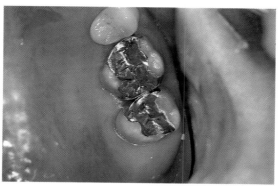

Fig. 209 Gold inlays in posterior teeth.

## Porcelain inlays/onlays

*Definition*

An intracoronal or onlay restoration made of porcelain (Fig. 210).

*Indications*

A posterior restoration where the major consideration is one of appearance.

*Advantages*

- The aesthetic result with these restorations can be very pleasing particularly when compared to amalgam (Figs 211 & 212).
- The use of resin-bonded techniques to lute these inlays/onlays in place means that this type will provide support and strengthen a weakened tooth, in contrast to a gold inlay.
- This restoration offers a viable alternative to more radical preparations such as crowning.

*Disadvantages*

- A porcelain inlay is more liable to fracture particularly if the margins are incorrectly prepared. Repair of the damaged restoration is difficult.
- These inlays also require the use of hydrofluoric acid to etch the fitting surface so that the luting cement will adhere to the porcelain. This etchant material has to be used in a fume cupboard and handled carefully.
- Adjustment of the occlusal profile of this restoration is difficult compared to other restorative materials.
- A porcelain inlay may produce excessive wear of the opposing tooth structure where there is parafunctional activity.

*Procedure*

- Castable ceramics can be used to fabricate the inlay on an investment model in the laboratory.
- Computer-aided design and fabrication techniques are now available so that the inlay can be machined from a block of porcelain.

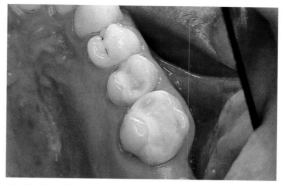

Fig. 210 Porcelain inlay.

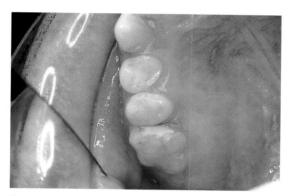

Fig. 211 Porcelain onlay preparations.

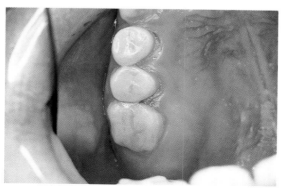

Fig. 212 Porcelain onlays cemented.

## Composite inlays

An intracoronal restoration fabricated from a composite resin material.

Restoration of a premolar tooth where the appearance may be compromised by other materials.

Apart from the aesthetic advantages previously mentioned, this type of inlay may be of benefit in a tooth that is more radically broken down and requires support before restoration can take place. Assuming sufficient enamel remains then resin bonding techniques are used to support the weakened tooth structure.

- The poor abrasion resistance of these restorations means that they are not suitable where there is parafunctional activity.
- They are not indicated in posterior teeth that carry excessive loads.

  This property of composite resins has restricted their use in the posterior regions of the mouth. Although the materials have improved and techniques for strengthening these materials have been developed, they still do not fulfil the criteria for an ideal posterior restorative material.

The cavity is prepared with a slightly increased internal taper than that for a gold inlay (Fig. 213). A gold inlay requires a 5° taper approximately while this is increased to around a 8–10° taper for a composite inlay. This is because the material is weaker and more liable to fracture prior to cementation (Figs 214 & 215).

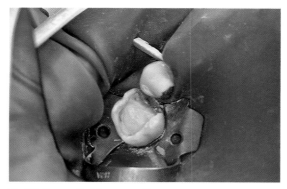

**Fig. 213** Composite inlay preparation.

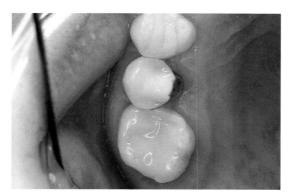

**Fig. 214** Composite inlay.

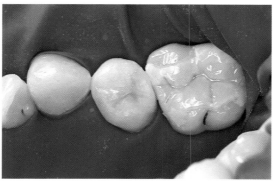

**Fig. 215** Composite inlay. (Courtesy of Dr A.C. Shortull)

## Subperiosteal implant

*Definitions*

- Implant with a removable superstructure.
- Cobalt/chromium casting that is inserted between the periosteum and the bone to support a denture (Fig. 216).

*History*

The first subperiosteal implant was placed by Dahl in Sweden in 1943 and this technique was employed until the early 1980s. The technique was slowly discontinued and replaced by blade–vent implants and subsequently by endosseous implants.

*Advantages*

This technique provided additional support and retention in an atrophic ridge situation. Whilst the implants had a reasonable success rate at five years, it dropped dramatically after this period.

*Disadvantages*

- The technique involved the taking of an impression of the underlying bone, necessitating a surgical procedure, and a subsequent procedure to place the metal casting.
- Bone resorption progressed and therefore these frameworks soon no longer fitted the underlying bone.
- Commonly infections tracked down the implant post causing infections in the underlying bone and exposure of the metal casting (Fig. 217).

*Procedure*

1. A surgical procedure was carried out to expose the bone and an impression of this was made.
2. This was then used to cast a cobalt/chromium framework which was placed under the periosteum; sometimes anchorage screws were placed to secure it to the underlying bone.
3. This was allowed to heal and a casting which had previously been made to fit the implant posts was incorporated into the denture base (Fig. 218).

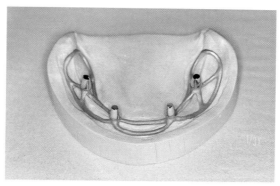

**Fig. 216** Subperiosteal implant structure.

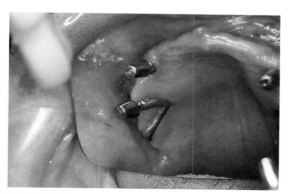

**Fig. 217** A failing maxillary subperiosteal implant.

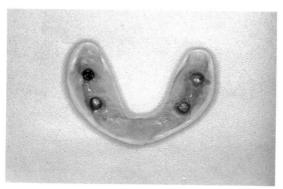

**Fig. 218** Fitting surface of overdenture.

# Dental implants and bar

*Definition*

A type of restoration where two to four implants are commonly placed in the edentulous arches and linked by a bar connector (Figs 219, 220 & 221).

*Indications*

An edentulous patient who has problems with the retention of complete dentures due to an inadequate ridge form.

*Advantages*

- The prosthetic treatment is straightforward. Therefore there is reduced time and expense when compared to other types of implant reconstruction.
- Fewer implants are required than for fixed implant prostheses and therefore treatment can be performed even if the bone availability is severely reduced.
- A removable prosthesis can compensate for defects in the ridge form as well as providing lip support.
- The patient's oral hygiene is simpler than for fixed implant prosthesis.
- The load is equally distributed between the implant fixtures.

*Disadvantages*

- Patients may object because the prosthesis is still removable.
- The prosthesis is mucosal borne and therefore regular checks are required for relining.
- The patient is still wearing a removable prosthesis and therefore the biting force and chewing efficiency is not that of a dentate individual.

*Procedure*

1. Impressions are taken of the fixtures and then either a direct or indirect technique is used to construct the bar.
2. This is then fabricated and tried in the mouth.
3. The overdenture is constructed in the normal manner and the clip is placed at the processing stage.

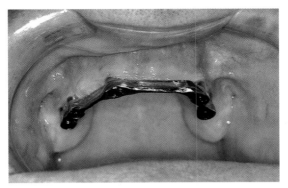

**Fig. 219** Maxillary bar for overdenture.

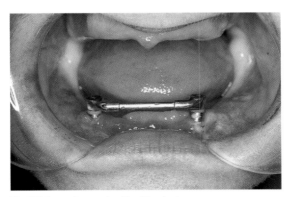

**Fig. 220** Lower bar retained by 2 implants.

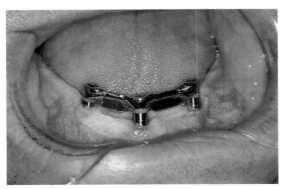

**Fig. 221** Lower bar retained by 3 implants.

## Implant and Hader bar in the reconstruction of a resection patient

*Definition*

Surgical excision of a tumour results commonly in an oral environment which is difficult to reconstruct. Implant placement can therefore provide added retention for the placement of a removable prosthesis (Figs 222, 223 & 224).

*Indications*

Patients who have had tumours resected often have problems with retention of prosthetic appliances. Even if the patient has had postoperative radiotherapy, implants can be placed under certain conditions.

*Advantages*

- The placement of implants can allow for retention of a large maxillofacial appliance which may not only replace the missing teeth but also the resected bony support as well.
- These appliances help in the rehabilitation of patients who have undergone a major traumatic experience.

*Disadvantages*

- Many patients who have had such radical surgery would prefer not to have further surgical episodes for the placement of implants.
- It may not always be possible to place implants around the resected site dependent on the quantity and quality of bone in that region.
- The use of implants in a region that has had radiotherapy may not be possible if certain criteria cannot be met.
- Implants can be placed within 6 months of radiotherapy or after hyperbaric oxygen treatment.

*Procedure*

The procedure is the same as previously outlined. However, it is also often beneficial to consider the use of a neutral zone technique when constructing the prosthesis, to determine the zone of minimal conflict for denture placement.

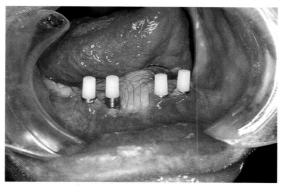

Fig. 222 Implants with impression copings in place.

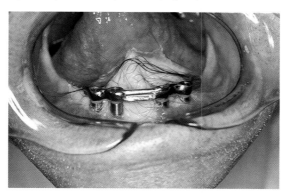

Fig. 223 Hader bar in a patient who has had a resection and radial forearm flap repair.

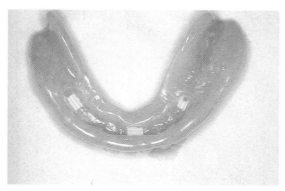

Fig. 224 Retentive clips in denture.

## Implants, bar and Ceka attachments in the management of a resection patient

*Method*

An overdenture normally attaches to an implant bar using a clip attachment, however it may be necessary to utilise other forms of retention (Fig. 225).

*Indications*

Where additional retention is required to attach the removable superstructure to the bar, attachments other than clips can be utilised (Fig. 226). The implants may have been placed so that insufficient space between the fixtures exists for a clip to be placed. The use of other smaller precision attachments can solve this problem (Fig. 227).

*Advantages*

- The dentures are retained by a resilient attachment to the bar and therefore no anteroposterior rocking associated with some designs of bar can occur.
- The attachment can be activated as and when wear of the component parts occurs rather than having to replace the clip or bar.

*Disadvantages*

- The additional cost of such attachments might be prohibitive.
- These attachments give a more rigid connection between the overdenture and implants and therefore the denture may potentially place more loading on the implant fixtures.

*Procedure*

The precision attachments are either cast or soldered into the bar during its construction stage.

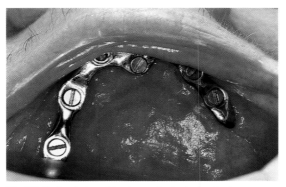

**Fig. 225** Occlusal view of bar in a patient who has had a resection.

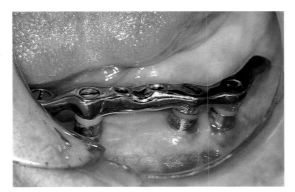

**Fig. 226** Implant with bar and Ceka attachments.

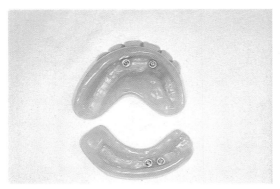

**Fig. 227** Fitting surface of overdentures.

# Magnets in implants

*Definition*

A metal alloy that possesses magnetic properties and therefore attracts a similar metal alloy.

*Indications*

This type of attachment offers an alternative to other implant systems (Fig. 228). It will result in a less obtrusive implant coronal surface in the mouth when compared to most other attachment methods (Fig. 229).

*Advantages*

- The housing is simply positioned within the denture base (Fig. 230).
- From a biomechanical viewpoint magnetic retention places virtually no force on the implants.

*Disadvantages*

- The magnets corrode with time and need replacement on a regular basis.
- This type of retention provides no lateral stability to the denture.

*Procedure*

The implant attachment is placed in the normal way and the magnet within its housing is cured into the denture base either in the laboratory or at the chairside.

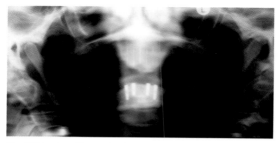

**Fig. 228** Implant fixtures in place.

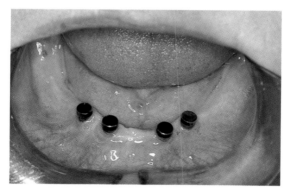

**Fig. 229** Magnet keepers on implant fixtures.

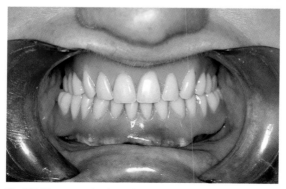

**Fig. 230** Magnet retained overdentures in place.

## Stud attachments

*Definition*

A system where the patrix component is attached to the implant and the matrix is housed within the denture base.

*Indications*

The placement of a stud attachment is one of personal choice (Figs 231 & 232). The indications for its use are the same as for that of bars and magnets (Fig. 233).

*Advantages*

The size of the attachment is smaller than a bar and therefore less room is required in the denture base. This may be of great benefit in a case where interocclusal clearance is limited.

*Disadvantages*

- The resilient 'washers' or 'O' rings perish with time and need to be replaced.
- They provide less retention than that of a bar.

*Procedure*

The patrix is attached to the implant and the matrix is placed within the denture base either at the processing stage or by using a direct technique at the chairside.

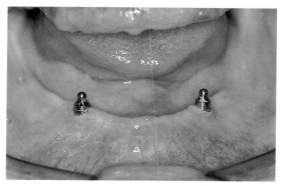

**Fig. 231** Studs placed on implant fixtures.

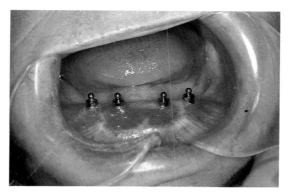

**Fig. 232** Four stud attachments on implant fixtures.

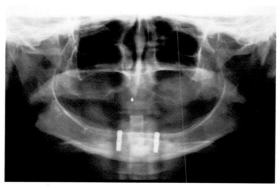

**Fig. 233** Radiographic appearance of implants.

### Single tooth implant (blade–vent)

*Definition*

A thin section of perforated titanium that is placed into the jaws and allowed to heal (Fig. 234).

*Indications*

When a tooth or multiple teeth were lost and a fixed or removable replacement was required without using the adjacent dentition. These implants were developed in the 1970s.

*Advantages*

- Because the implants were flat in cross-section, the width of remaining bone was irrelevant.
- The placement procedure was easy to perform.

*Disadvantages*

Many of these implants failed to integrate with bone and were kept in place by fibrous scar tissue. Whilst this allowed the implants to function for many years, they often became infected.

*Procedure*

1. A full thickness flap is reflected and the crestal bone is exposed.
2. A bur is used to cut a channel and any debris is removed.
3. The implant is placed in the slot and tapped until the shoulder is level with the crestal bone.
4. The flap is replaced with multiple sutures and the area allowed to heal.
5. The superstructure is constructed after a suitable period for healing (Figs 235 & 236).

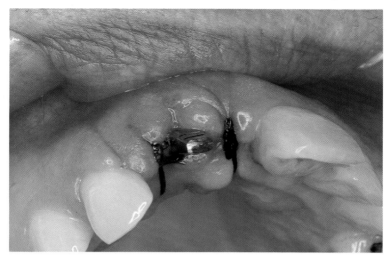

**Fig. 234** Blade-vent implant.

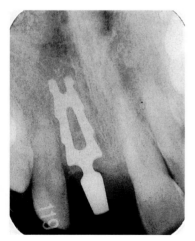

**Fig. 235** Radiographic appearance.

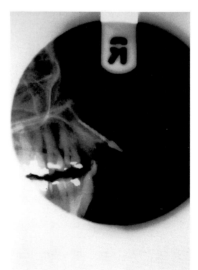

**Fig. 236** Lateral view showing angulation of blade-vent implant.

# Single tooth implant

*Definition*

**Tubingen (Frialet–1)** (Figs 237 & 238)
A ceramic artificial root that can osseointegrate to replace a single missing unit.

*Indications*

Where an immediate implant placement system is needed. If a tooth requires extraction and an implant replacement is viable then both procedures can be done in the same visit.

*Advantages*

- This implant is described as an 'open' implant in the sense that the coronal portion is exposed during the healing period: only one surgical stage is required.
- The ceramic nature of the implant means that the margin can be prepared with an air rotor to provide the desired margin.

*Disadvantages*

Success rates of this implant system are poorer than for other systems because:
- the implant might be placed in a socket that is still infected, and therefore a delayed placement technique is advocated;
- the implant material itself is brittle and liable to fracture;
- the success of osseointegration seems to be less than that of titanium implant systems.

*Procedure*

1. The tooth root is extracted as atraumatically as possible, the socket is prepared, and this single stage implant fixture is placed (Fig. 239).
2. A temporary restoration is placed to protect the implant from loading during the healing phase.
3. An impression is then taken after integration for the superstructure to be constructed and finally cemented.

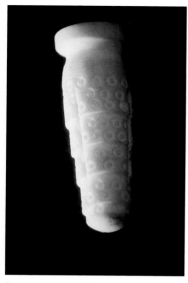

**Fig. 237** Frialet-1 (Tubingen) ceramic implant.

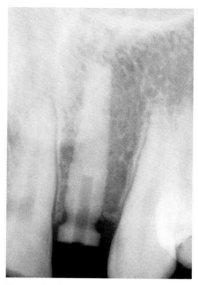

**Fig. 238** Radiographic appearance.

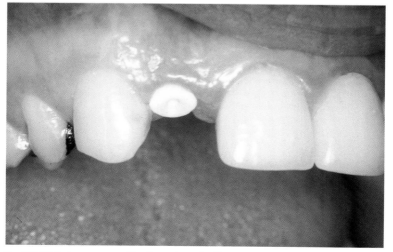

**Fig. 239** Clinical appearance of implant prior to loading.

# Single tooth implant

*Definition*

**Branemark (Cera-one abutment)** (Fig. 240)
A titanium implant fixture used to replace a single tooth.

*Indications*

Where sufficient bone (height and width) exists for the placement of the implant fixture. Where a tooth has been lost but the supporting bone is still adequate and the neighbouring teeth are sound and the occlusion favourable.

*Advantages*

- Adjacent teeth do not require preparation for use as abutments for resin-retained bridgework.
- Good appearance can be achieved and the proximal surfaces can be cleaned easily.

*Disadvantages*

- Surgery is required.
- The placement of an implant may not be possible if there is inadequate bone or if anatomical structures or occlusal relationships are unfavourable.

*Procedure*

1. The implant is placed using an internal coolant drill so that the bone does not overheat.
2. It is covered over and allowed to integrate for a period of between three and six months.
3. The Branemark single tooth system allows for several types of connection to this abutment, which can be either cemented or screw-retained (Figs 241 & 242).

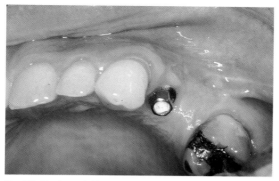

**Fig. 240** Single tooth Branemark implant in place.

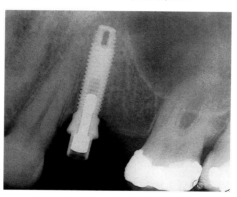

**Fig. 241** Radiographic appearance showing superstructure to be fully seated.

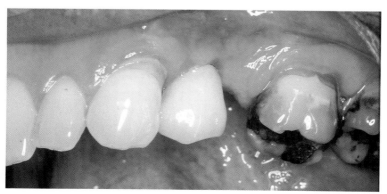

**Fig. 242** Single ceramic crown replacement using a Branemark implant.

# Maxillary implants with acrylic bridgework (IMZ)

*Definition*

A rigid prosthesis that is nonremovable by the patient and is supported purely by the implants.

*Indications*

Where adequate bone exists for the placement of multiple implants and both the functional and therapeutic benefits are considered to be greater than those of a removable implant-borne prosthesis.

*Advantages*

- There is clearly increased stability of the restoration when compared to a removable appliance and the load is evenly distributed amongst the implant fixtures.
- There is no direct contact of the prosthesis to the alveolar mucosa therefore no forces are transmitted to the crestal bone. Alveolar resorption is likely to be reduced.

*Disadvantages*

- Phonetic, functional and aesthetic problems may result because of the height of the superstructure in relation to the residual ridge.
- Oral hygiene is more difficult to maintain since the appliance is not removable.

*Procedure*

1. An impression is taken of the implant fixtures and a casting constructed to determine that the fit is good around all the implant fixtures (Fig. 243).
2. The acrylic superstructure is then processed onto this bar by conventional techniques (Figs 244 & 245).

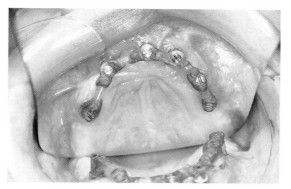

**Fig. 243** Try-in of duralay bar prior to superstructure being cast.

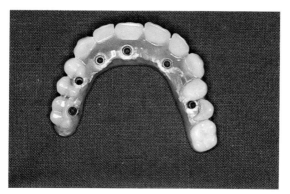

**Fig. 244** Acrylic fixed superstructure.

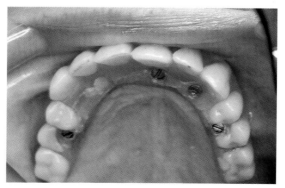

**Fig. 245** Occlusal view of fixed implant retained bridge in place.

## Mandibular implants in a resection patient with acrylic bridgework (IMZ)

*Definition*

Fixed bridgework that has been rigidly fixed to several implants (Figs 246 & 247).

*Indications*

This type of prosthesis is indicated in a patient who has had a mandibular resection and reconstruction using, for example, a radial forearm flap. The construction of a conventional prosthesis or even a removable implant-borne prosthesis for such a patient may be unsatisfactory for many reasons, including loss of sensation and muscle tone of that region. Therefore the placement of a fixed prosthesis in this case provides many benefits.

*Advantages*

- The prosthesis is stable and can be tolerated even although the normal architecture of the region may have been destroyed by the ablative surgery.
- The fact that the patient can eat and talk as normal after such radical surgery has psychological as well as functional benefits.

*Method*

- If a flap containing skin has been used to repair the surgical site it is advisable to reduce the thickness of the tissue prior to placing the implant superstructure.
- A graft is placed around the necks of the implants with oral epithelium, as skin does not provide a suitable gingival collar for an implant.

*Procedure*

1. The implants are placed using a surgical stent to locate the implant fixture in the ideal position.
2. The implant is left unloaded to integrate.
3. Impressions are taken and the superstructure constructed in the normal manner (Fig. 248).

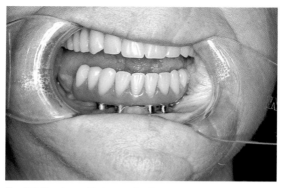

**Fig. 246** Fixed mandibular prosthesis.

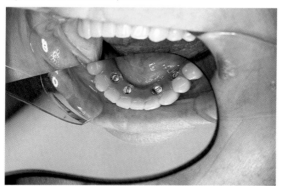

**Fig. 247** Occlusal view of fixed prosthesis showing screw attachments.

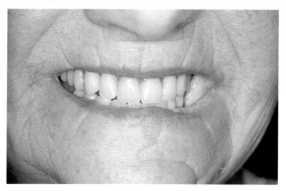

**Fig. 248** Finished result of a complete upper denture opposed by a fixed implant bridge.

# Implants with fixed bridgework (Astra)

*Definition*

- Implants with a fixed superstructure.
- The placement of several implants to provide support for fixed bridgework (Fig. 249).

*Indications*

- Where multiple tooth units have been lost and sufficient height and width of bone exists for the placement of implants.
- Where sufficient interocclusal clearance is present to allow for subsequent implant superstructure placement.

*Advantages*

- The metal superstructure can be cast in one piece instead of multiple single units.
- The splinting of two adjacent crowns should provide better load distribution.
- Linking multiple implant units resolves rotation problems, overcome by other implant systems by having internal coronal hexagons.

*Disadvantages*

The occlusion of fixed implant bridgework must be adjusted so that the implant-borne crowns are adjusted to be about 0.1 mm out of occlusion to avoid overloading during maximal intercuspation.

This is still an area of much debate as is the question of the best method of linking implant and natural tooth units.

*Procedure*

1. The implants are placed in the conventional manner and allowed to integrate.
2. The porcelain-bonded superstructure is constructed and fastened onto the implants using screw attachments (Fig. 250).
3. The occlusion should be checked and refined carefully (Fig. 251).

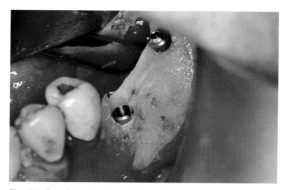

**Fig. 249** Two Astra implants at time of insertion.

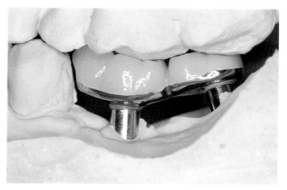

**Fig. 250** Laboratory construction of porcelain fixed superstructure.

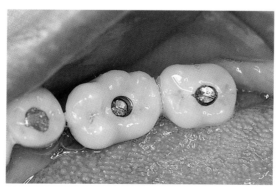

**Fig. 251** Completed bridgework in place.

# Index